"A beautifully written testimony to the human spirit and its capacity when stretched to its limits… Should be on the reading list for all those involved in cancer care." *Dr Elspeth Salter, Centre Head, Clinical Psychologist, Maggie's Fife*

"Excellent reading for health care professionals, medical and nursing students and anyone touched by cancer." *Professor Marie Fallon, St Columba's Hospice Chair of Palliative Medicine, University of Edinburgh*

"A remarkably beautiful and powerful account [that] will be of great help to others dealing with the ongoing challenges of cancer care." *Andy Anderson, Maggie's Edinburgh, Centre Head*

"[Clark] lights a fire at the heart of the story, a flame of human warmth that keeps burning however harrowing the events become." *Jamie Jauncey, author*

"Reading the book has helped reinforce some of the reasons why doctors such as myself do the job… it can make a difference to people's lives." *Duncan McLaren, oncologist*

"A searingly honest, compelling account [which] makes valuable, and sometimes difficult, reading for doctors about what really matters to people facing such a challenge… The unrelenting progression of the disease and the intensity of the suffering may engender unease and apprehension in the reader. The couple's response to it engenders, more strongly, respect and admiration for the human spirit." *Dr. Lesley Morrison*

The following reviews were ᵥ   *rt's*
'CancerVoices'. They are not t   *rt.*

"This is ɑ   ɩe neart."
Prostate

"Compelling and articulate... offers a powerful insight into the range of emotions experienced and some strategies for protection and self-preservation. It will help those with cancer and [their carers] by offering a connection with others who have been through the experience... [and] a toolbox of ideas for those currently on their cancer journey. I recommend this book across the board." *Cancer survivor, former oncology nurse*

"A truly inspirational read and very useful, particularly for carers, friends and relatives... It is a pleasure to read and incredibly difficult to put down! This has to be added to my list of best books ever read. Absolute top marks for this amazing book." *Breast cancer patient*

"This account is not appropriate for every stage of cancer... [but] if you have no illusions, it might dramatically improve your strategy and confidence; it is rich in advice, humour, hope, strategy and love... It is a fantastic example of learning through experience and using this learning to help others." *Breast cancer survivor*

"Deals frankly with many issues, including end of life. It is most useful for carers and should be read by cancer health professionals. I suggest that patients wait until after treatment to read it." *Survivor of leukaemia*

"I read it in two days and wish I had read it 10 years ago." *Living with breast cancer & relative of bladder cancer patient*

'Excellent in helping the reader feel that they are not alone with the cancer nightmare... If you are not a fluffy, pink-ribbon person and need a more down-to-earth approach, this book provides an excellent, truthful approach... [but] it is at times harrowing." *Living with breast cancer*

CELLMATES

Our lessons in cancer, life, love and loss

Rose T. Clark

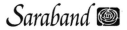

Saraband

Published by Saraband
Suite 202, 98 Woodlands Road
Glasgow, G3 6HB, Scotland
www.saraband.net

ISBN: 978-190864317-9
ebook: 978-190864324-7

Printed in the EU on paper from sustainably managed sources.

1   3   5   7   9   10   8   6   4   2

To me it's ironic that the smallest unit of life within us, the clever building blocks that allow us to be healthy human beings, can alter and divide out of control into an inhumane threat to any one of us at any time. They are the Jekyll and Hyde of our physiology.

please note
The author wrote this powerful personal account primarily to raise awareness of critical issues relating to cancer care. The intended audiences are medical professionals and policymakers, but it may also be appropriate for some patients in palliative care and their carers, as well as those recently bereaved. The language is sometimes graphic and the sections covering pain management may be disturbing, particularly to recently diagnosed patients or those with a recurrence of their disease.

If you are a patient or carer, please seek appropriate advice and resources to help you at your particular stage of diagnosis and treatment. Organisations dedicated to helping you through cancer and bereavement are listed at the back of this book.

*For the many people who dedicate their time to caring for others.
It is not until you are in the hands of your knowledge and instincts
that you realise the enormity of what you do. With your help John
and I were able to live in times of true happiness. We remember you
and thank you for making a difference each day.*

Duncan McLaren
Marie Fallon
Claire Hunter, Elliot Longworth, Joan Scott, Tara Mulube and
    all the staff at John's local medical practice
Elspeth Salter, Andy Anderson and all the staff at Maggie's
    Edinburgh
John MacFarlane
The nurses and doctors from the first floor Marie Curie
    Hospice Fairmilehead, Edinburgh
The nurses, doctors and consultants at the Western General
    Hospital Oncology Wards and Chemotherapy Day Unit
The district nurses, Marie Curie nurses – especially Eleanor –
    and those from the Nursing Guild who sensitively helped
    care for John in our home
Macmillan Cancer Care
The nurses, physiotherapists and consultants at the Edinburgh
    Royal Infirmary

contents

cell [biology]
The smallest structural and functional unit of an organism
Oxford English Dictionary

cancer [mass noun]
A disease caused by an uncontrolled division of abnormal cells into part of the body
Oxford English Dictionary

foreword

Professor Marie Fallon
St Columba's Hospice Chair of Palliative Medicine,
Edinburgh Cancer Centre and University of Edinburgh

Although I see patients with incurable illness every day and I like
to think I understand a lot about what people endure, I was surprised by the impact of Rose's story. This is a beautifully written
book. It is firstly the story of two people who love each other
and the journey, at times tumultuous, of that love story. Alongside this very personal, honest and touching account of their love
is the struggle with cancer and all that it encompasses for both
John, as patient, and Rose, as partner and carer.

This is an account of hope, despair, highs, lows and, of course,
challenges with the health care system and at times with individuals within that system. The account of all these aspects is told in
a very integrated and human way; nothing is in isolation, rather
it is part of a bigger picture which is both very personal and very
honest. For these reasons I think this is an outstanding read for all
health care professionals, both postgraduate and undergraduate.
We talk about 'integrated care' but rarely about 'integrated outcomes'. Rose gives a very vivid account, which is multifaceted

and multidimensional, of two very real people. It is a picture that no professional could ever build from reading a textbook or even an in-depth discussion at consultation.

However, this story, which at times can be happy, warm and comforting, and at other times distressing, is more than anything a beautifully crafted, sensitively told and startlingly honest account of the lives of two people. The general reader will find they cannot put it down.

If you are reading this foreword and you have cancer or someone close to you has cancer, I would say that if you like an honest, straightforward approach, then you might draw help from this book. There are tips on how to deal with problems and situations, but more than anything you may draw from the account of Rose and John's relationship and, in particular, Rose's ability to articulate her feelings.

This book is a powerful gem: profound, honest, a love story, a journey through cancer, told in a compelling way.

why it is important to read this

Dr Elspeth Salter
Centre Head / Clinical Psychologist, Maggie's Fife

Any reader opening the covers of *Cellmates* will be taken to the heart of Rose and John's relationship and the gruelling experience they shared of John's cancer. It is a beautifully written testimony to the human spirit when stretched to its limits. The remarkably frank honesty of the writing presents a truly challenging read, no matter how experienced you are in the field of cancer care or of human suffering. But I encourage the reader to continue reading, even through tears, because this is both an enlightening and inspiring human story.

I truly believe this book should be on the reading list for all those involved professionally in cancer care. Anyone working or considering working professionally in the field of cancer would do well to read this extraordinary and powerful personal account. You will discover what matters most to patients and their loved ones as they face life's ultimate challenge. The sense of tender love shared and tested in the midst of a very human struggle with pain and fear is expressed with vivid realism. The account highlights the importance and value of a variety of sources of support for couples facing a terminal diagnosis and the need at times for an outlet for the tensions felt in even the most loving of relationships as the strain of the struggle tells.

Read with care but read on if you are in a similar position to Rose and John. Rose writes beautifully but without sentimentality. She honestly shares with you the reality of her experience. She will inspire you and offer you practical guidance. If you are caring for a loved one or have lost someone to cancer then this book will challenge you but also offer important routes to supporting yourself and giving yourself permission to struggle at times. Rose's experience of accessing support later than she felt was ideal will hopefully encourage you to take the step through the door of services like those of the Maggie's Centre to get whatever help you may need, practical or emotional, and to recognise the resources you have within yourself to deal with each new challenge one day at a time.

It was a privilege to get to know Rose as she did all she could to support John. She continues to support him as she fulfils his wishes in publishing this extraordinary and truly remarkable account of their shared experience and embarks on her continuing story. As a Clinical Psychologist I strive to embrace a sense of human resilience and to offer permission for human emotion in the face of serious challenges in life – this book succeeds in both. It will encourage others caring for someone with an incurable cancer and it will inspire all of us who fear cancer that there is a way through even such a daunting challenge.

part one
the cancer

I watch your chest rise and fall, rise and fall, and then it stops. It's only seconds I think, just seems longer, more like minutes. I know it's going to happen but I'm not scared. Why am I not scared? Why does it not feel wrong? For the first time in months you are peaceful. And so am I. Tears come to me but I just watch you lying there. Dying.

In this moment I want you to die. This must be wrong? I love you, I'm scared to be without you, I don't know who I am when we are not trapped in this cell together, fighting to get out. My purpose is to keep you here, to make it better. But I can't keep watching you like this. We are too broken, too tired. It must end. This must be it, the end. It's strangely peaceful but I heard it might be this way; after all the pain and struggle, it might be a gentle release. We've been here before, exhausted, aware of the odds, preparing ourselves for the inevitable. We come back, we always do. It becomes our joke it's so unbelievable.

The comfort starts to seep out of me, my calm, accepting mind drowned out by mounting panic, thudding in my chest, burning skin. It's not happening, it can't be. I can't let you go, not ever. I put my hand on your chest and whisper: 'are you still with me?' You say something, but it's not me you are talking to. Wherever you are, you are not here. You look serene, happy, pain-free. But I panic. I'm selfish and my heart is clawing at me to keep you. I shout at you and shake you and make you be here. You finally come round. You look barely conscious but then you start to look confused, realisation spreading across your face. Something has happened that has scared you and you begin to sob uncontrollably. I comfort you, saying it's going to be ok, that we always get through. You're inconsolable in a way I have never seen you before. I know that you've gone somewhere which makes you feel differently; your stubborn feet are not so securely planted on this earth.

To this day I wonder if I had left you looking that peaceful, your face relaxed not strained with pain, if that would have been the end. And I feel guilty because I brought you back. I thought I was bringing you back to my love and care, and for your strong, proud body to stand tall again. But what lay ahead, how could we know. It was months before you took your last breath. The most tragic, most happy, most exhausting, most defining few months of my life.

I'm Rose. John and I shared nearly eight years of our lives together. For the last three years of our relationship, cancer anchored us together. That's not as grim as it might sound.

This is our story. A story of how two ordinary people live with the diagnosis, the check-ups, the disappointments, the relief, the questions, the answers, the operations, the recovery, the emergencies, the denial, the acceptance, the anger, the pain, the loss, the love, the fear, the frustration and the happiness.

We are scarred by what I think of as 'the talons of cancer'. The things that claw into you, securing a hold deep under your skin, leaving you constantly wriggling to break free. The most suspensive of these is the pendulum between despair and hope. Eventually, we learned not to fight against the swing of the pendulum. We grew to accept that we needed to live with the cancer, to stop trying to maintain normal routines and meet expectations. We dealt with each new difficulty as it unfolded, in the day we were in. We treasured the good times, developed a profound level of closeness and found fulfilment in simple things. We achieved what you rarely attain in good health. We ran from death, and in doing so found life.

I was often so consumed in mechanically surviving that I couldn't tell John or anyone else how I felt. So I wrote letters to John and diary entries to no one, none of it meant for reading. When he found these John asked me to share them with others, to release the realities of a subject muffled by white coats and a fear of knowing. As I tell our story I share some of these letters and entries. They are our truth, not our act.

My words are to raise awareness of the challenges faced by those with cancer and the loved ones caring for them. I am aware that professionals dedicated to cancer care can become burdened by pressures on their time and resources. Growing patient numbers, inadequate staffing levels and facilities, restrictive financial budgets; the cold economic and political factors which increasingly dictate the treatment of cancer in our society. Yet human honesty can be enough to remind all of us what matters most to the people behind the labels of 'patient' and 'carer'. For this reason I write with unflinching honesty, sometimes graphic and distressing, so we may truly address subjects such as care at home, pain management and the vital role of charity-funded support organisations. These sections of the book may be upsetting particularly to those people in the early stages of cancer treatment so if you are in such a position please consider whether this book is appropriate for you.

We learned a lot during our experience of cancer, much of it I wish we had known earlier. Simple practical tips and more significant emotional observations which helped us to breathe in life alongside the cancer. I know our story is fast-paced so at the end of the book I remind you of things that aided us.

If it helps even one person to deal with the challenges of cancer and caring for someone with it, if it helps one medical professional relate to patients and their relatives then this book is worth writing.

The moustache and the mink bathroom

What was my initial thought the first time I met the man I would fight unconditionally for? 'What a dodgy moustache.' Yes, that was definitely my first overwhelming thought. 'Very smartly turned out, stands tall and proud, handsome broad shoulders, immaculate, yes, ex-army I'd guess, but that moustache, get out of the eighties, man.' Then: 'big smile, think it's genuine, but lord you're gonna crush my fingers with that handshake, wow, you mean business man-with-the-dodgy-moustache, you're telling me you are who you are and you're not going to shy away from it.'

As it turned out I wasn't too far wrong. He was fiercely proud and was ex-army. He joined the army at 16 in August 1975, completed two years apprenticeship then six years service as a mechanic, mainly with the Scots Guard Second Battalion.

My first meeting with John was 4 April 2002 in a lounge at the George Hotel in Edinburgh. My solicitor had recommended that I go to John's firm to arrange a mortgage. Neither of us was on great form. I was going through a divorce, decidedly drained, bedraggled and wound up. John's girlfriend had just died. He was utterly devastated in a way I would not understand until later in my life. He was still, however, remarkably together – on the surface that is.

The meeting set in motion a deep friendship. John was 42 and I was 27. He looked a bit younger, I looked a bit older. We had both weathered a few adventures, good and bad, some chosen, some not. We had both made mistakes and achievements and were both annoyingly stubborn. Neither of us was usually the type to let our guard down but that first meeting happened at a time when we were raw and open. John talked about his girlfriend, about his two daughters (from earlier relationships), about his business and his friends. He did not talk about his cancer diagnosis, not because he was avoiding it but because he did not, would not, entertain it. He was invincible even in his bereaved state. Most people who met John realised quickly that, whatever his past and scars, he was a man of admirable strength and courage.

We talked for a long time that first meeting until rumbling stomachs and buzzing phone messages woke us from our mutual therapy session. As we walked out of the hotel and along George Street John insisted on walking on the traffic side of the pavement. Somehow this unselfconscious gesture took on an outsize significance for me: it seemed the icing on the broad-shoulders, firm-handshake, door-held-open and shiny-shoes cake. He may be by some accounts – mostly true – a bit of a lad from Fife but he was also a gentleman.

During the weeks that followed, our emails and calls gradually and naturally increased. It was as if, after unwittingly showing our vulnerability to each other and realising that neither of us was able to admit weakness to friends or family, we needed to check the other one was doing ok. Eventually, when all my business dealings with John were over, he asked if he could take me out to lunch to say thanks for all my thoughtful checking on him. I remember discussing with female colleagues what exactly the invitation meant: was it purely friends, should I refuse the invitation despite feeling increasingly close to this troubled but intriguing man with the dodgy moustache. They all advised me to decline the invitation. So of course I said yes.

We were to meet on Friday 2 August 2002 at my favourite fish restaurant. We hadn't actually seen each other for a while, the friendship fuelled mainly by emails and phone calls. When I met him he said: 'You're a lot prettier than I remember.' As he was a man of brutal honesty I was rather chuffed but I said: 'You say it as if it's a problem', to which he replied: 'It could be.'

Friends or more than that, it was a great date. We talked and laughed, enjoyed tasty food and guzzled two bottles of Chablis. When John said I wasn't to worry about his intentions as he couldn't date a client, I replied that he wasn't to worry about mine as I could never date a man with a dodgy moustache. It must have been the Chablis that made me agree to help John renovate his bathroom. After I told him about the renovations I was doing to my flat he admitted his mink bathroom suite might be in need of the skip, and his yellow and green walls in need of white emulsion. He in turn agreed to hang a heavy oak mirror in my lounge. And so it was that we set date two.

The following Saturday I opened my door to greet my friend with the dodgy moustache. He was there smiling in a slightly nervous and suggestive way. The moustache was no longer. And there the trouble began. I never envisaged Victor Paris as the main stage for romantic involvement, but it was. The mink bathroom suite actually survived until John sold his cottage, securing in my mum's head at least that it was all a clever ploy. Thank goodness I did not tell her about his fridge full of Chablis and fresh strawberries on the first day I viewed the ugliest bathroom in Scotland.

You have to dive deep for the best lobsters

We relaxed surprisingly quickly into a relationship. At first it was hidden to the outside world. John had his cottage in Fife, I had my flat in Edinburgh. Mostly we would hang out at my place, and in no time at all John was staying over most nights. We talked a lot, sitting at the dinner table for several hours discussing everything under the sun. It was very us, something we did right till the end. It's what I miss most.

We went on some great trips but the most special were spent at Loch Tay. We were both captivated by this vast water with the imposing Ben Lawers watching over it. We would walk for hours in layer after layer of dense forest, wander round Taymouth Castle and always end days huddled in a corner of the hotel in the pretty white-washed village of Kenmore, which sits at the outflow of the loch to the River Tay. One of our favourite memories was a magical snowy New Year in the village square, eating from the outdoor barbecue, drinking beer and watching fireworks crackle above the fairytale church. John was at his happiest, most relaxed, most free on these trips.

Our beloved Loch Tay was not responsible for the nickname that became cemented like no other. John became known as Lobster, or later Lobby or Lobs, after a winter holiday to Tenerife in 2003. It was a throw-away comment: 'Are you sure you want to go abroad with me? One day of sun and I'll resemble a giant freckled lobster.' It just stuck. To begin with he was embarrassed by his Lobster persona but he soon embraced it after I pointed out that it reflected his hard outer shell and killer claws protecting a sought-after delicacy within... and I loved 'getting away with' calling him by his cartoon persona in public.

The only time we spent apart was for work, John's golf, my running, and of course John's weekends with his daughters (who were with their mums during the week and every second weekend), of which I was terrified in the early days. We kept our contentment quiet. Our friends were understandably nervous about us entering a new relationship. It took some friends a long time to relax with us being a couple.

I waited several months before I agreed to meet John's girls; they were pre-school and primary school ages at the time. I remember the day clearly: utter terror is hard to forget. But after ten minutes I knew it would be fine. The youngest was a charming cutie with the most endearing freckles, while the eldest was clever, funny, sharp and unmistakably John. We laughed at John's story telling of all the daft naughty things 'dad John' had done. I knew how much John loved his children but seeing them together and listening to the love and laughter really touched me. It also scared me a little. I was definitely the outsider and I would have to be very careful not to try to force myself into their lives, just be there, as someone who loved their dad, and let them come to me. I started to hang out with them on the weekends and grew to love them. John was in his element cooking them roast dinners and being a rock for them. When it came to parental matters, John was firm but fair – everything he did and said was to protect them and make them learn how to be self-sufficient and confident. He was also fun. I will never forget how hearty the girls' laughter was in response to their dad's nonsense.

Looking back, the first two years of our relationship were really happy. But soon living between two homes became tiring and impractical. It was time for us to 'make or break', as John put it. We were either together as a family or not, and if we were we needed to buy a house together. I was not at all ready to find myself in a four-bedroom house with a garden and garage and most importantly two kids. I was jittery about the whole move, teetering on the edge of changing my mind. But I knew John and I should have a chance to be together; there was always an undeniable pull I could not quite understand. And so it was that I agreed to turn my life upside down, inside out, for the giant freckled Lobster.

A good par three

When we were looking for places to live there were three important factors. Number one, a good golf course for John. Two, I needed to see hills and trees. Three, the house had to be big enough to be a family home, room for the kids to feel settled when they stayed with us and for me to hide when I needed to. It did not take us long to settle on a conservation village in the Scottish Borders that has a beautiful golf course and is surrounded on all sides by glorious rolling hills.

We bought the house in November 2004 and, after I subjected it to an internal transformation, we moved into it in the spring of 2005. John loved the place. He walked around it, admiring the view, enjoying the peace and often said he felt he was finally home. We had barbecues with the girls and played Pictionary till late in the night. John climbed ladders, chopped wood, mowed the grass, rebuilt drystane dykes, cooked his magical roast dinners and golfed, golfed, golfed. When he was at home he was relaxed, something he found hard to do generally. We were lucky to feel such contentment, even if we did not realise it at the time.

We had a lot of fun in 2004. My 30th birthday was in September and we dragged out the celebrations for weeks. While I was juggling the logistics of getting the keys to our new house and organising plumbers and painters, John jetted off to Thailand with his golfing friends. John was exuberant that year; he was attacking life at full force, the only way he knew how, and loving every minute of it. Finding our new home fuelled his energy but so too did news that he had long awaited – his cancer was very unlikely to return.

A near miss, a far certainty

John's first experience of cancer was in 1998. A routine medical discovered blood in his urine. The doctors confirmed a diagnosis of bladder cancer in September that year, the day after John and his business partner Paul opened the doors of their new financial services firm in Edinburgh.

The cancer was a transitional cell carcinoma of the bladder graded as G3, the highest grading, meaning that the cells look very abnormal and are most likely to quickly grow and spread. As the cancer had reached the stage of invading the bladder wall it was classed as T2. If the cancer is only in the innermost lining of the bladder it's referred to as carcinoma in situ, but when it progresses further into the bladder it's categorised with a rating of between T1 and T4. John had been diagnosed with invasive bladder cancer.

The specialists told John that if he did not have his bladder removed, plus parts of the surrounding organs, his chances of surviving more than five years were less than 50%. John was 39 years old, active, proud and exceptionally stubborn. And having a second daughter only a couple of months old, who was with him at the appointment, meant he had no intention of having his quality of life impaired to such an extent. Instead of surgery John and his oncologist Duncan agreed to radical radiotherapy. The treatment worked and in July 2004, with no reoccurrence of the disease, the guidance was that the cancer was unlikely to reappear.

We breathed a huge sigh of relief. Well, actually that is not true, because I'm not sure I was ever concerned that it would come back. John was an indestructible character and never showed any worry that the disease would re-enter his life. He had defied the doctors' expectations once, so he was sure that his mind-over-matter approach could cure anything. I believed him.

The day I first realised John had been quietly worried was the day his younger daughter began school – a year earlier. The day a child starts school is a special day for any parent, but for John this day was especially significant. When he was first diagnosed with bladder cancer in 1998 a specialist told him that he was very unlikely to see his younger daughter start school. From that moment on John had made some decisions based on the fact he would only live five years. He looked up old friends, he cancelled his pension and he took up golf. So, while on the surface he refused to entertain talk of cancer, underneath it was eating away at him. The sight of John's younger daughter that day would have brought happy tears to anyone's eyes: all excitement and apprehension, cute freckles and red hair, cheeky smiles and wide eyes and, like her father, too fiercely proud to show what she was feeling. I'll never forget John calling me from his car after she walked through the school gates. He was not crying, he was sobbing. This was not a man provoked easily to tears so I was quite taken aback. He was sobbing with utter relief. Deep down part of him had feared he would not see that day, and he suddenly realised he had everything to live for.

In a startling moment that same day I thought a weird karma of sorts was at work – it looked as though John's just realised joy was to be snuffed out in some cruel stab of fate. Driving to John's cottage in Fife, we stopped at a local shop. John turned to say something to me as he took his first steps to cross the road. I remember a screaming horn and then John's face turning pale with horror. He was somewhere else in that moment, lost in the relief of the day, and walked straight out in front of a car. We were thankful for the quick reactions of the driver as we quietly considered the meaning of the moment.

I respect the uncertainty, the cruelty of fate. The giving one minute, the taking the next. I felt that day was a warning to pay attention, to live in the moment, to appreciate what we had. When John was given the all clear by the hospital the following year it was the last piece of the psychological jigsaw in place allowing him to really relax into his new life in the Borders countryside.

I was right about fate.

Confessions of a golfer

We found out the cancer was back on one of John's golf days. When John was diagnosed with bladder cancer in 1998 golf was on his 'bucket list'; boy did he commit himself to that decision with zeal bordering on somewhat irritating obsession. As his 'other half' I feel permitted to confess that John was a major golf bore. At one time early in our relationship he even talked me into getting golf lessons so we could enjoy, or at least go on, golf holidays together. I tried, I really did. But my encouraging start in the driving range did not translate well onto green or fairway, preferring to settle stubbornly in the rough. Having to think about the position of my feet, legs, back, arms, neck, the projection of a perfect swing, and at the end of it try to hit a ridiculously small ball with an only marginally larger bat was too much. In the end I confessed to John I'd much rather just walk round with him and be his caddy.

Even the player/caddy partnership was not always a perfect marriage. I quickly learnt that John was a stickler for course rules, written and unwritten. The day he hit a ball off a tree and I burst out laughing was the day I realised one had to carefully manage one's automatic responses on a golf course. The day I was designated buggy driver on holiday and drank too many vodka and cranberry juices in my stationary moments I realised one must pay absolute attention to keeping the score card and not, ever, tell the player he's lining up a drive for a par three instead of a par five. It was a most sombre drive to the next hole and marred my enthusiasm for the outstanding idea of a refreshment buggy on a course.

Although John was proud of his own strength he was later mortified about how he handled things the day he was told cancer cells were returning to his bladder wall. The cell change was discovered at a routine check-up at a hospital in Dunfermline. The consultant wanted to act quickly and suggested a cystoscopy, a procedure involving a probe to burn away the cancer cells with an electric current. John, as usual, had planned his day with precision and was due to play golf with his friend Ken that afternoon. In his wisdom, or lack of it, John decided to go ahead with the game – after part of the lining of his bladder had been burnt away. He called me at work after the treatment to explain what had been said. I remember sitting at my desk and feeling the floor fall away from under me. I felt sick, and the warmth drained from me. It was one of the most marked responses I felt to all the news we received after John's check-ups, though it was way down the list in terms of severity. I think it was because it was the first time I genuinely realised that the cancer was a threat, that it could come back and burst our bubble. I didn't absorb the words 'I'm still going to play golf' – they were ridiculous after all – until I later repeated them in my head over and over in growing frustration and anger. So while John struggled his way round 18 holes, yes he bloody well played the full round, I found myself crying in a loo in work and then disappearing home. When John finally joined me he looked dreadful and was in a lot of discomfort. Although we later laughed with friends about John's typical iron man behaviour he was in bad shape by the end of that day. He really could not understand my upset or concern for him. It was the first, tiny step in John realising that what happened to him and how he behaved had a huge impact on the people he loved and who loved him.

Foreigners in a new world
Once I knew the bladder cancer was on the prowl I began researching everything I could find out about it. Information was and continued to be my way of dealing with the uncertainty. The more I knew about the disease and treatments the better able I was to tackle it like some sort of project. If I was informed then I was more prepared to fight for John, to ask the questions, to explain the responses. I never thought I knew better than anyone else; my priority was to know what to ask the professionals.

I wish we had discovered earlier in our forced exploration of cancer about how to work as a team, especially when dealing with consultants and hospital procedures. As you go along you learn the short cuts and techniques to make sure you get attention when you really need it. Hospitals are an alien environment for the novice patient not helped by the fact that the medical profession seem to work in hostile silos. Different departments within the same building appear cut off by continents and if your treatments span more than one hospital then you had better be on the ball and make sure they are talking to each other. But I will return to that later.

One thing we discovered quickly was that John would shut off in appointments with his oncologist or consultants, especially if he was receiving bad news. Often he would come out of appointments with little or no recollection of what had been said. When we recognised this we began preparing better for appointments and check-ups: John would explain to me what he wanted to know and we would agree a list of questions. John had trouble articulating how he felt and I almost acted like a translator for him. I focused my attention in the appointment, often writing down the doctors' responses in the session or just after. That night we would go over it again and note down any research we wanted to do to better understand medical terms or options. The other practical benefit of me accompanying John to his appointments was to detail his symptoms to the doctors. If he was unwell after a treatment he would often not remember what had happened and could not give doctors the key information they required about symptoms and side effects. When things became graver, John would have hours and days missing from his memory, either because he was not fully conscious at the time or because his mind was blocking out the potency of the pain. I learnt to record any physical, mental and emotional changes I saw in John; it was a useful way to notice what was a definite change and to stop justifying everything as a general ache and pain. Of course with cancer in the room the genuinely innocent aches and pains become a source of worry and a feeling of vulnerability.

We were quite a pair for displays of bravado but when I look back I realise that even in the early stages of the cancer's return the worry of its potential course was cementing an underlying stress in our lives. By Christmas that year we knew that the cancer cells were on the attack again. A small operation was scheduled for the beginning of 2006. We decided not to tell our families or friends until after Christmas and New Year. I remember my family spending Christmas with us and John and I feeling frazzled. The demands of work, the kids, preparing to host Christmas, all glued together with niggling uncertainty created two tired and tetchy individuals. John began staying up late at nights listening to music. I'd go to bed early then wake up in the early hours to find I was alone in bed. I'd go back downstairs to find John lying sound asleep in one of his favourite black squishy chairs with Pink Floyd, David Bowie, Coldplay or some obscure artist galloping through his subconscious. Alongside golf, music was John's next favourite hobby. He would shut himself in a cocoon of music for several hours every night until I dragged him up to bed where he would deliver a chorus of snoring in seconds while I lay awake wondering what he was thinking and feeling. My family tells me we carried Christmas off without them suspecting a thing, but I knew of the late-night arguments between John and me, the type of tired bickering that comes from pestering uncertainty. John was drumming out his worry by working non-stop either at his office or at the house, exerting himself physically with endless outdoor chores. I was worried sick that he was pushing himself too hard at a time he needed to give his body rest. We followed Christmas with a three-day trip to Barcelona on 13 January, to celebrate my mum's 60th birthday. An enjoyable few days filled with sightseeing, good food and too much wine, though we struggled to keep the pace. Of course we worked hard not to show it. As we bounced our way up the hundreds of steps at the Sagrada Familia, to everyone else we looked as if not a worry rested on our shoulders.

I refer to uncertainty a lot. It is by far the worst 'talon' cancer sank into us, especially in the early days when we were learning the ropes that swung wildly off the side of its treacherous precipice. None of us really know what waits round the corner despite how hard we might plan or work or protect but we tend not to focus on our vulnerability. When cancer is the known relative we refuse to talk about, in the hope that it never rejoins the family, the picture of your future is somehow dirtied. Certain dreams you have or hopes for the future begin to falter a little. You dare not make some plans in case it tempts fate into humbling you yet further.

The fact the cancer had come back at all frayed our tough denial. But the more I understood about the cancer the more I convinced myself it would all be ok. The cancer was contained in John's bladder, it had not breached the wall, therefore it was not en route to other organs. If the doctors had dealt with it once, they could deal with it again. John's resolve to beat it was untouchable and mine was not far off. Although the uncertainty was crawling under our skin we would not tolerate the continuation of this disease in our lives. On that we agreed and we were invincible in our joint defence. I also focused on the advancement of cancer treatments, the trials and breakthroughs I kept reading about. New drugs that did not exist when John was first diagnosed could now be a lifeline. Surely science could outrun John's cancer. In 2006 we would embrace such a treatment with open arms, excited by its simplicity, its irony, glad it was as an option.

Fighting fire with fire

In February John went for a minor operation to remove the cancer cells that had reappeared. They were caught at an early stage and classed as carcinoma in situ. The consultant explained that after the operation John would be sent for immunotherapy treatments to try to prevent the cancer from progressing into invasive cancer.

All we knew initially was that the immunotherapy was to begin at the end of March and was to use the living bacterial vaccine BCG for tuberculosis inserted into the bladder via a catheter. We were both slightly frightened and intrigued by the idea; it sounded ludicrous to begin with. However, the theory seemed wonderfully simple. In slightly crude terms, our understanding was that if you introduce a disease into your body, which your immune system recognises as damaging, it will automatically fight to get rid of it. So if you apply these foreign bacteria into the bladder the immune system will fight to overcome the disease by increasing white blood cells and attacking cancer cells. At first when we began researching BCG treatments we couldn't find very much in the UK. Most of the available research papers we could find were from the US. The research suggested that doctors were not exactly sure how the BCG treatments work but the results for treating early bladder cancers were encouraging. John loved learning about this surprising treatment and telling friends about it, gory details and all.

On Wednesday 29 March, I took John to a private hospital in Edinburgh, thanks to my company healthcare cover, for the first of six treatments. I was to collect him a few hours later once the procedure was over. I found it hard to believe it was actual BCG, diluted or not, that was being inserted into John's bladder until we were told that John was not to have contact with pregnant women for two days after the treatment and we were to put bleach down the toilet every time John passed urine.

The first treatment lulled us into a false sense of security. While it was exceptionally uncomfortable for John – as he put it: 'that hole is designed for fluid to come out of it, not a ruddy great tube inserted up it' – he seemed fine afterwards. Some hot sweats, slight discomfort peeing but nothing too worrying. John's immune system was actually impressively good. I know that may sound strange, as he was fighting a deadly disease, but he did show it who was boss for a long period, and in between times standard colds, tummy upsets, the flu would unsettle him for a day at most. If he did show signs of catching something he'd sweat it out overnight and be marching through life the next day as normal. He did not 'do' unwell and had little tolerance for anyone around him being sniffly, sweaty, pale or weak-willed. Not always a good character trait but he never pretended otherwise. John's enviable immunity meant that when the doctors began feeding the BCG into his bladder his system leapt straight into action and began a counter attack with force. The treatment was predominantly used on older patients, those with less robust immune function, and it took several treatments at a high dose to jolt their systems into fight.

By his third treatment John's body was firmly focused on barging the unwelcome visitor out of his system by shedding his bladder wall. It was agonising for John. 'That hole' is most certainly not designed for passing anything solid through it. We quickly came to dread each Wednesday. The effect of the treatment was cumulative and John would be in a worsening state after each one. I spent the night holding him over the toilet while he screamed in agony trying to pass his body's triumphant removal of the foreign threat. The doctors were delighted; the treatment was working. John's bladder was killing off the BCG and as a happy result the cancer cells with it. The doctors stopped the first batch of treatments before we completed them as John's response was so marked and as, quite honestly, he couldn't take any more. It was an arduous few weeks but if it worked it was acceptable to us.

The next batch of three BCG treatments was scheduled for September, and John set out to have fun that summer before he endured more pain. We kicked off with the village's annual summer festival. In Aberdeenshire, in the village I grew up in, we had a one-day fair each year. In the Scottish Borders they take things a little more seriously. The festival stems from traditions of horsemanship and it involves difficult rideouts through the local hills, sporting events, competitions, and a lot of partying. We were invited to a 'wanna be' fancy dress party. John didn't do fancy dress. A man of pressed trousers, starched shirts, shiny shoes and cufflinks was difficult to get into full-blown superhero/popstar/sportsman gear. The best I could do was talk him into wearing a huge pair of angel wings and a fluffy white halo while I donned devil horns, tail and a trident. The rather loose link was John 'wanted to be more angelic' and I 'wanted to be more devilish'.

I need not have worried about our lack of commitment to the costumes as the sight of John in wings and a fluffy halo raised smiles from those who knew him well. He was still tired after his treatments but he launched into the night, the beers, and the wine, with gusto while I danced the night away with similar, slightly disillusioned gusto. (John did not dance, not ever, even at weddings – well, apart from in the privacy of our kitchen, and it was more a slow swaying cuddle to music than a dance.) Much of that night is a blur but I do recall leaning John over my shoulder to drag him along the one mile walk home from the village, up a long steadily rising incline. At our sides were our wonderful neighbours Bill and Ann, who on that night were the Man from Del Monte and Suzie Quatro. It was no wonder the passing cars tipped their full beam back on to do a double take at this staggering motley crew.

I managed to get John up the stairs, undressed and into bed. It was not the first time I did this, and certainly not the last. John was not one to shy away from a night out, whether he felt well or not. On one occasion I found him slumped in the corridor of a hotel in full highland dress, legs akimbo with nothing left to the imagination. He had made it back to the hotel but swiping the door key card was too much to navigate. If the giggles of an American couple hadn't woke me he would have slept soundly there until the morning breakfast trollies rattled past him. There were many more good days and nights out which ended with him sleeping like a baby. John tackled alcohol like he tackled illness: he kept going till he keeled over, slept it off then bounced up the next day as if nothing had happened.

Shortly after our summer festival capers we headed to my brother's in the Peak District for a couple of days. It was after a day walking there that I realised that John's resilient front was hiding a struggling body. His pride meant that at no point did he say he'd had enough, despite my asking. He didn't want my brother to think that he was in any way weakened by the cancer or the treatment. I still look at a photo taken on that trip and see his weary eyes staring back at me. It catches my breath and sickens me; why did he push so hard?

John always kept a page from an old desk calendar in his diary; it has a quote on it that reads: 'Have the courage to live. Anyone can die.' This was John's essence: he was never, no matter how bad things got, dying. Every minute that would allow, and some tried damn hard not to, John would live it to the full. Unless John was asleep or unconscious he was firing on all cylinders, and everyone around him knew it.

We followed the trip to my brother's with a gloriously sunny week in Prague. Sightseeing, admiring the Gothic architecture and lazing in outdoor cafes and bars perked John up before his second set of treatments began in September. He endured the nasty side effects and we got through it. Although worn physically, John kept his foot firmly on the pedal. I knew there was no point in stopping him so I went along for the ride and prayed the road ahead would be kinder to us. I was becoming an increasingly nervous passenger. I felt trapped in this out-of-control cage watching my life fly past on the outside. John did not get angry at the cancer, instead venting his frustration on those minor annoyances that don't really matter: car drivers not indicating, shoppers not saying thank you when he opened a door for them, queue jumpers. He began obsessing over controlling everything around him, in his office, in the car or in the house. He had a precise way of doing each task, and his way was the only way he accepted. I began to understand that this was because he could not change the really big thing in our life so he compensated by trying to control everything else. I knew he needed to talk to someone about the cancer and how he felt, but he refused. For now I was absorbing the fallout and trying not to take the mood swings and verbal aggression personally. It wore me down. Every trip in the car, every post-day analysis over dinner became an assault to my ears and a weight on my heart. The only way I managed to keep my mouth shut and protect myself was to remember why this angry person had taken residence inside my Lobster. I knew why he sat up late each night hiding in his musical universe, but I needed him to face the mental and emotional pain in the real world, alongside me.

I was glad when John went on his annual golf trip to Tenerife in the November of that year. We both needed a break. The only people we spoke to openly about the cancer were each other. When we looked into the other's eyes, even on good days, the truth stared back at us. Sometimes we just needed to forget, to step back into our normal worlds with friends and colleagues where the cancer was rarely mentioned. I worried of course, as I always did when I was not with John, but it was fine and he returned looking terrible but having had a ball. The next set of BCG treatments began on Thursday 29 March 2007. Before that John managed to squeeze in a quick trip to Dublin with his friends from Fife for St Patrick's Day. Again, he came back looking terrible but having had a ball. I knew he was packing in the good stuff to take his mind off the bad stuff.

We both dreaded the treatment beginning but refrained from dwelling on it and did not waste time moaning about something that was a necessity. We would do anything to keep the cancer at bay and we felt strong in our resolve to do so. But there is always a limit. I knew within a couple of hours of collecting John from the hospital that they had taken the treatment too far. John's temperature shot up, he was shaking, lightheaded, nauseous and had a rash. He could barely stand to go to the toilet, and when he did manage to do so, the pain would buckle his legs under him. I got John to bed and we muddled slowly through the night, with me carrying John back and forth to the toilet and trying to keep his temperature down. He settled fairly quickly over the next couple of days but I made sure we expressed our concern to the consultant about John's intense reaction to the latest BCG treatment.

Easter number one
The next treatment was on Thursday 5 April, the day before Good Friday. I wish we had not gone. I remember picking John up from the hospital and getting him home. It was a beautiful spring evening and we settled in the conservatory to eat a meal. John was sore but always liked to sit at a table to eat. I voiced my concern. He insisted. I made him one of his favourite comfort meals: chicken kiev, cauliflower and mashed potato. He gave up after a couple of mouthfuls; he was feeling sick and lightheaded and was burning up. I lifted him up from his seat but his legs went from under him. I don't clearly remember what happened next

but I know I got him back and forth from the sofa to the down-stairs toilet a couple of times. He was shaking violently. The pain when he passed urine was worse than it had ever been; he was screaming, crying with exhaustion and frustration. The last time I took him to the toilet we managed to prop him up between the wall and the sink and he asked me to go and get him some water and a painkiller, which I did. I should have stayed with him.

I heard him fall, and when I got through the doors I knew he was unconscious. I tried to pull him up into the recovery position but he was too heavy and jammed in the small room. I ran out of the house and hammered on Bill and Ann's door. Bill looked horri-fied when I said John had collapsed. The two of us managed to get John up on his feet and onto the sofa and at some point he became conscious again. Bill sat with John while I called the ambulance and explained the treatment he had had that day. I asked if he could be taken back to the private hospital or the oncology wards at the Western, where his oncologist was based, but I was told he would need to go to a large general hospital with no specialist cancer unit. I knew this was madness even then, as the staff at this hospital would not know about John's cancer or the treatment, or have an oncologist on call to see John. A first responder arrived within minutes. She turned out to be a neighbour from down the road and I felt immediate relief at her arrival. I talked her through the treatment and what had happened since we got home, told her that I believed that the BCG dose had been too high for John to take and he had passed out due to pain. After Bill and one of our local firemen redirected the lost ambulance to our home, the ambulance crew settled John with painkillers and ran through with me again what had happened. John was quickly en route to the hospital while I followed in my car.

The accident and emergency department was like a club 18–30 holiday night gone wrong. It was Easter holiday week-end and most of Edinburgh and the Lothians seemed to have drunk themselves into a sick stupor or a nasty accident. John was stretchered in and left in a corridor to be seen by a doctor. I was told to report to reception and then wait in the general waiting room until I was called. It was mobbed and I found it impossible to sit face to face with people sporting minor, mainly drink-related, injuries when I feared John was in a lot of trouble. I'm not sure how long I forced myself to maintain a polite position in the fume-filled room but every minute of following hospital procedure gnawed at my willpower, and even more so at my instincts. I needed to be with John. I was right. When I found him to my total horror he was still in a corridor, barely conscious, choking on his own vomit. I sat him up and turned him on his side. To anyone else among the throng of patients and harassed doctors I guess he looked like another drunk gone wrong. I was angry. I walked round into the main A&E treatment area, grabbed a doctor's arm and told him firmly that the man choking on his own vomit in the corridor had cancer and had collapsed at home following an immunotherapy BCG treatment inserted into his bladder that day. Somehow, to my surprise, the stress did not confuse or upset me; it enhanced my purpose and clarity. I knew that in order to get John seen I must convey the problem without antagonising already stressed doctors. Within minutes we had another doctor at our side, who listened to my summary of John's medical history, treatments and details of his appointed oncologist and consultants.

We were moved into a curtained-off room in the main A&E department where we were confined for hours. It was a relief to have John on machines that could warn of a change, it was a relief to be close to medicines and doctors. It was not a relief to be in the wrong hospital. They treated John's pain and gave him fluids, but I did not know why we were there. They could not get hold of the consultant who was in charge of John's BCG treatments and they could not get hold of his oncologist. It was what I grew to call 'the Easter effect' – an unpleasant attachment we seemed unable to shake off in subsequent years. It was holiday weekend, most of the doctors and consultants were off. The unlucky ones attending were dealing with the dregs of many a bottle.

We were in that sodding room for hours. I sat in a hard plastic chair next to John and waited for various nurses and doctors coming in to ask the same questions that a colleague had asked an hour earlier. But I knew they were just doing a job, a job that involves too many patients, too few beds, too few staff, long hours and mostly not a lot of thanks. When I ventured out to get a cup of water I felt humbled by the work the medical staff do. The place was overrun with genuine cases of broken bones and sickness but also the aftermath of a good night out and even a wedding: half a congregation seemed to be sitting at the side of one bed, high heels, chiffon dresses and fascinators looking ridiculously comedic in the sterile surroundings.

After many hours of wrangling between hospitals it was agreed that John would be moved by ambulance to the Western, where his oncologist would see him the next day. This was what I wanted, needed, to hear – that we would soon be in the safe and knowledgeable hands of Duncan. In the early hours of the morning John was transferred to a general ward there, as there were no beds in the oncology wards. It struck me that the ambulance drivers were glad to talk to two people who were neither drunk nor threatening to assault them. It's easy to ignore a world until you fall into it. I have the utmost respect for the people who look after us when we fall ill or injured. They may well feel rewarded when they help deserving people but they have an enormous amount of unacceptable shit to deal with.

By 3am John was settled in a bed in an out-of-the-way ward with no other patients in it. The silence was a relief. I tried to sleep in yet another hard chair (can no one design a reasonably priced but comfortable NHS chair?) next to John, but couldn't. I started to throw up at this point, something I later learned was my body's standard reaction to too much adrenalin and not enough sleep. A nurse recommended that I go home and come back in the morning. Home was eighteen miles away and I was not safe to drive. I had plenty of friends who lived close by but I worried about waking them in the middle of the night and I didn't want to have to explain to anyone – again – what had happened. After unsuccessful attempts at sleeping on various inhospitable chairs and in my car, which was too cold, I felt a bit sorry for myself. My cropped trousers and thin t-shirt were not assisting my comfort levels. I had been focused on packing a bag for John when the ambulance drivers had arrived at the house, not on preparing myself for a night sleeping rough. In the end I found myself at a hotel a couple of streets away, explaining my situation and asking for a room for a few hours. They gave me one, for next to no money. It failed to bring me much sleep but I was glad of the warm soft bed cradling me. In the morning I made a cup of tea and ate the complementary shortbread to fill my stomach. When I got to the hospital John had been moved to an oncology bed and after a wait we saw the welcome face of Duncan. We were in the right place, with the best person. Relief.

That was the end of the BCG treatments, and as it turned out they had done their job. John's bladder was clear. Of course, as John regaled the story to friends and family, his favourite bit was showing them the nasty-looking burn mark on his left leg. As effective as my crisis management had been there was some room for improvement. When I ran next door to get help I left John's leg propped against the steel towel rail in the toilet, which I hadn't noticed was on. John couldn't recall how he developed this ugly reaction/mark/injury on his leg, a mystery that caused the nurses and doctors confusion. It wasn't until later when I was describing events in detail to John that we realised what had happened. When we checked, his burn matched exactly the width of the radiator's steel bars. I was mortified. He was endlessly amused.

Despite our teasing it had been a traumatic experience, the first time either of us was properly scared. The first time I considered I could lose John. But we survived it, and the treatments, however unpleasant, did their job. I also realise that during that episode I gained insight that would better arm me to tackle what lay ahead. I now knew at which point John would lose consciousness due to pain or weakness, what colour and temperature his skin would be, how much his shaking would intensify. I knew how to speed up the process of collection in an ambulance and admission to a hospital. I typed up a sheet containing the key points of his medical history, the contact details of his oncologist, and our doctor, which I updated with his current medications. I'd hand this to the first responder, the ambulance driver, the admissions doctor – it's what they need to know and stops the endless questions. I wrote down the direct numbers of all the wards and departments I might need to get through to in a hurry. I realised we needed to shout louder when we felt a treatment was having side effects that might be dangerous. I could pack a bag quickly with everything John needed and liked for his stay, plus his notes and medications – it takes time to get prescriptions in the hospital. I knew it was sometimes better to call our 'out-of-hours' doctor's service to see us through the night until we could be admitted to the right hospital in the morning. I knew what to say, to whom, when to be hard and when to gently appeal to someone to make sure John received care. It had been a steep learning curve but this newfound knowledge made a big difference to how I handled the progression of John's illness. It also helped me develop a good relationship with most of the medical professionals we came to know. They could see I wanted to help John and that I understood and appreciated what they were doing for him. I saw the challenges they face within a hospital system that tries its best but often fails to feel human. It is a different world, one all of us hope we will never enter on the patient side, never rely on. Like everything else you have to adapt to your surroundings, whether you like them or not, to get the best out of them.

The check-ups following Easter gave John some comfort. He at least knew the pain had been worth it. He recovered quickly and bounced back into life. I remember him cooking a roast dinner for friends only a couple of days after he was out of hospital. I tried to cancel; he was irritated by the suggestion. I didn't have the cheek to tell him that actually I was emotionally and physically drained and would rather not face socialising. Although John was still in considerable discomfort and was exhausted he donned his apron and smiling host face to turn out an impressive turkey joint and perfectly roasted potatoes. He was quite something. No wonder most people close to us thought John was indestructible.

I did not feel the same; the cancer was always out there whatever the weather, no matter how bright the forecast. It was beginning to turn life into a slog. I failed to get the same relief after check-ups. Instead of feeling joy at positive news I felt defeated and sad. I spoke of this confusion in my first letter to John, my way of talking to him without him hearing. He found it in a hidden folder on my computer.

I am glad, Lobby, that today we can mark off another checkup. These are intense, frustrating landmarks which blight a month or more with anguished build-up: uncertainty, hope, fears and in the end just bloody submission to whatever God decides is inevitable. At some point you just give in to fate I guess. No matter how much you worry or pray, offering to sacrifice one thing for the desired outcome, it makes no difference. I always find that the week before your check-ups is exhausting emotionally and physically. I can see you growing more anxious by the day. It starts with a few quick words and a distant look in your eyes and grows to a remarkable pretence that everything will be ok. I suppose we both pretend a lot — if we did not, how would others around us cope?

Today produced the best outcome we could hope for and I could see in your eyes the relief, perhaps not so much that it had not eaten back into you but that all that pain, inflicted by some supposed treatment, had not been in vain. But when the consultant told me that all was well, that you had responded, and even that, going forward, this cruel but necessary treatment may be lessened, all I could feel was a relentless sadness. Something I could not explain to myself let alone to you or anyone else.

You see, it never truly goes away, it lurks like some foreboding presence over our future. It might be a longer-term holiday booking, a change of jobs, or property plan, or my deep unattainable dream to one day have children in the face of this persistent shit of a disease. No matter what it is, this damned thing is bearing down over our staunch and proud shoulders.

I hope to wake tomorrow and feel the relief that our friends and family do. The relief that for a while it can be forgotten about, that daily life can go on and we can worry about getting to work and faulty washing machines. To forget for a time that life is so very precious and deeply unfair. I have often said that you will beat this cancer and make the rest of us feel humble in doing so. But I know that by some cruel twist of fate, a remarkably unnecessary and easily avoidable incident will take your honourable life from us. I know this because that is the way life works. We all fight long and hard to stay here, sometimes against the hardest of odds, but in the end, we are so easily snuffed out like some incidental amusement in the greater scheme of things. So perhaps this realisation is where my sadness lies today, why I can't look into your eyes and say it is great, we can enjoy life for a while. When I have seen you in such basic, raw, inhumane pain it is difficult to believe this. I can't forget the last treatment, it haunts me today as it did then: the desperate feeling of helplessness, the disgusting loss of control, the bare fear that I might lose you through pure ignorance of the situation.

We were very alone during the last treatment. Like brave but naive children, who were prepared to do what they were told. We are both proud and determined to tackle what is thrown our way. But even people like us get scared. By the third treatment I was terrified. When I saw you, the person I love and respect, the person who is my anchor and foundation, crumble under real physical pain, it was a humbling experience. When it looks as if you may

lose the strongest person you know, it makes you fear for yourself.
Being the woman of a brave, stubborn man is never easy. Being
the woman of a brave, stubborn man fighting something relentless
and deadly leaves you worn. But I can't tell you this; it is not you
to look at things in this way. I will continue to stand quietly by
your side.

John found the letter one night when he was listening to music,
whiling away the hours until sleep rescued him. He didn't talk
to me about it straight away. We had another big fall-out, initi-
ated by John's irrational road rage. I was angry and beaten low
by the demands of work and John's health. Why did this man
whom I had turned my life upside down for, whom I supported
without question, act with such unnecessary anger, talk in such
harsh tones to those closest to him, obsess over stuff that did
not matter, refuse to tackle his thoughts and emotions over the
actual problem staring us in the face? I was becoming tired of
supporting his hostility. I wanted to help him, I knew how to, but
he would not accept that he needed help. We hadn't spoken properly for days – something that had never happened before and
never did again – when he came and told me he'd read the letter.
He was crying, in realisation that people close to him loved him
enough to be scared about losing him. He hadn't stopped to think
how I felt, watching him suffer. The letter helped. We changed as
a couple, things got better, calmer. Until the cancer came back.

A change of scenery

I'm not sure when I began cycling but I remember spending a lot
of hours during 2006 and 2007 pedalling. My best friends Gill
and Nik got me hooked after a visit to Glentress, a local moun-
tain-biking haven of thrilling tracks through the forest. I visited
Glentress several times before settling for the less suicidal turf of

the Pentland hills, a stone's throw from my front door. I am notoriously clumsy, and my friends and John breathed a sigh of relief at my more sedate choice. Cycling became my escape. I pedalled out the anger, the fear, the loss of control. I was using John's bike, which was too big for me and hurt my back, but so what. At the weekends I set off on routes over the Pentland hills and came back exhilarated, covered in mud and cow poo and beaming the happiest smile John said he had ever seen on my face. I've always felt most at home in the countryside and love to trudge across hills whatever the weather, but cycling seemed freer. It kept me balanced. At this point I didn't consider the cancer a real threat to anywhere except John's bladder. I was struggling much more with John's anger and my absorption of it. My work was also getting me down; I had been there too long and could not see a clear path of progression that appealed to me. I felt trapped on all sides. John could see this and agreed that now was as good a time as any for me to start looking at positions with other companies. His health was settled, the scan results were clear and we felt confident we would not face big problems in the short term.

Before I looked at changing jobs, we decided to go to the Algarve for a week's holiday in May 2007 to give John a break from all the aggravations around him and me a break from hearing about them. I was keen to maintain my fitness by walking and running on the beach. We were in a resort near Alvor and the spot was perfect: our apartment was three levels up, right on the beach, built into a curved rock face. It had a glorious outlook framed by the dramatic rock faces typical of the Algarve. We had superb fish restaurants on either side: one in a neighbouring cove, casual, perfect for daytime lounging, the other on our right, a bit more special for an evening meal. We ate freshly caught, simply cooked fish of the day, salads, all washed down with bottles of Planalto, our favourite Portuguese wine at the time. John relaxed and began to look well and strong. He was keen to do a bit of exercise and I was nagging him to join me on my daily morning hike along the beach and back, about six miles. John always grumbled when I dragged him out walking; he was happy to cover miles if he was pulling a golf buggy, otherwise he wasn't interested. He blamed it on being forced out on endless, arduous hikes over cold, wet moors when he was in the army. So when, on our first walk together, he grumbled about niggling pain in his right leg I put it down to reluctance more than anything else. When he tried again the next day and the pain seemed worse we decided he should leave the walking be. The beach was on an angle after all and if he'd pulled something, walking on an incline would aggravate it. In some ways I was not surprised. John was determined to live life at 100 miles an hour, to work long hours, to play golf when his body was tired, to climb ladders, to cut grass, to fix guttering. Of course aches and pains would appear.

When we were in the Algarve that week, away from the interference of work, families, hassles, it felt like John and me again. We were happy. But it was only days later that the stress and frustration returned to John, and to me. His leg was niggling at him, his business was facing tough times and he was working longer hours. Weekends with the kids were difficult; we tried to keep up a front, to protect them from reality, but by the end of it John was always exhausted. The cracks were reappearing and we worried they could sense it.

In relationship terms 2007 was a year we would rather forget. We grew apart significantly. The cosy chats after dinner stopped, and when they did happen ended in arguments. When John lost his temper or overreacted I no longer sat quietly until it was over; I shouted back at him and told him he was being irrational and that the cancer was the cause of his anger, not other people. I begged him to get help, to talk to someone about it but his pride always answered no. It was truly horrible. We had been through such a lot together but the strain of doing so now caused us to push each other away. I was hurt by John's refusal to get help, his seeming willingness to keep taking it out on me instead. I rebelled against his bullying and resented the situation I was in. I had turned my life upside down to live his family life, to look after him and help him pretend to his children and friends that everything was fine when it was not. I had sacrificed my own opportunities at work and with friends. I loved him, I didn't mind this weight for a second, until his own anger began to drain me of my life in a way that others could see. The cancer was affecting more than just John's body; it was changing how he dealt with people, and the harder we tried to ignore its presence the worse the situation became. I began spending more time with friends and on nights out, and having feelings for someone else who said the right things, the nice things I needed to hear.

If ever John and I were close to splitting up it was in the summer of 2007. I couldn't honestly see a way back. After a horrible drive home when John had pursued a ridiculous road rage incident to an almost tragic conclusion I decided I had reached my limit. I calmly told him I could not carry on the way we were, I cared for him unconditionally, but that I deserved better, that I wanted it to end. John was horrified that I had reached the point of leaving. He knew I must be at breaking point to say such a thing. He tried hard to convince me to stay. I did, despite what my head was telling me. It was not a magical resolution; we were distant to each other, protecting ourselves from further hurt. John knew we were withdrawing from each other but later told me he felt we both needed space after the trauma of the previous year. He hated that the treatments had put such pressure on me and that I was living a life older than my years. I know now that John was trying to push me away to protect me. Like everything else in our lives, our purpose as a couple could not be controlled by either one of us. We were always anchored together even when we sat on opposite poles.

When it came to taking John's two girls on holiday in July we decided it would be best if John went on his own with them. Things were tense between us and I was increasingly feeling like an outsider when I was with them. I knew how much we had been through and we thought it best to hide most of it from the children, rightly or wrongly. But this meant always putting on an act and me carrying the situation along as if everything was normal. The pretence just took its toll. John and the girls had a great week's holiday in the Costa del Sol and I was glad I had not encroached on this special time. I felt relief at having a week to myself with no anger, tension or uncertainty. It made me realise that John and I had to make or break soon. When John returned from holiday he was complaining of worsening pain in his right hip and thigh. He went to the doctor, but all the signs pointed to nerve pain, so he was referred for some specialist massage, which relieved the pain for a few hours until it came back stronger than ever.

Around the same time I managed to secure a job offer. It was an exciting opportunity for me to progress, though I was warned that it would be a demanding role requiring stamina, enthusiasm and a thick skin. I needed a personal challenge, something just for me, and John encouraged and supported me in accepting the job. I began the new job on 20 August. The first couple of weeks were overwhelming. I realised the extent of what I had to set up and the limitations of the resources. The hours were long and overcrowded but I felt alive, confident and excited about the future. Despite the increasing pain in his leg John was genuinely happy to see things looking brighter for me personally. Our chats after dinner resumed, more animated and passionate than ever. We were settling back into us again and it felt right, meant to be.

I think I was into my fourth week at the new job when the doctor sent John for an X-ray. It was only a matter of hours before the hospital contacted our local surgery, which then called John at work to ask if a doctor could visit us at home that same evening. We knew something uncomfortable was about to unfold before us. But we had been here before, so a stiff upper lip and disregard to reality held us together. Inside we were both in sickening turmoil but we would not let this show to the doctor, to a man we had not met. It was a difficult thing for this young doctor to be faced with – to have to deliver worrying news to a couple he did not know. He looked nervous when he arrived at the house and as I showed him to a seat at our kitchen table I felt sorry for him. John and I were almost hardened to hearing such news, and John's inappropriate sense of humour in the face of awkwardness only fuelled the unease. I'm not sure what our new doctor expected us to say when he told us that John had cancer in his right hip and femur but I suspect we held it together quite well. I think we were wearing our masks again: 'Well, we showed the bladder cancer who's boss, we'll be able to defeat a bit of cancer in the hip no problem.' Our new doctor was called Elliot and he would grow to know us better, to see the couple behind the bravado.

After Elliot left, we were not so self-controlled. John broke down completely. He asked how we would get through it again. He said I should leave him now, that I didn't deserve any more of this shit and more of his stress. I remember quite clearly how I felt as Elliot delivered the news. I was defiant and decisive. The fog of past stress, of differences and bickering disappeared, and I was left with my truth. The cancer would not break us, it would make us stronger. I told John that I knew we had grown apart, that we were close to being over, but now on that evening I knew without question that I was meant to be with him. That we were a team who would fight this, that the fact that we were complete opposites in every way meant that together we had the tools to keep life in our hands. I felt and meant every word I said to John, and from that day on we both made sure we kept close enough that the cancer, and other people, did not wriggle between us. By my telling John that I would stand by his side no matter what, he was able to let down some barriers and let in some love.

Letter to John, Tuesday 18 September 2007

Each of us has pushed the other away. Perhaps together the reality, the uncertainty of it, was real and impossible to ignore. With others we could pretend, imagine ourselves before what we've seen, replace the fear with optimism about the future and be confident in who we believe we are and will be. I know you don't see yourself as someone who is ill, who depends on another. I understand your anger but I can't absorb it any longer. You are crushing me with your vocal aggression, exhausting me with your relentless picking and confrontation. You target this confusion at the most inane, unimportant things. You invite more stress into our lives, you actively pursue it. I see beyond your protective barriers to the complication of hurt from your past, to the fear of the cancer whether you admit it or not. Your anger at others, at minor mistakes, comes from this threat inside you. You pretend the cancer does not affect you, so what is this you do? Why would you ignore the one thing that can harm you and those you love in favour of pointless destruction? I can be patient, I can listen and coax you to momentary peace but we need help to stop this disease taking your mind and emotion as well as your body. You accept the help we need to protect your machine but you won't look after its precious drivers.

I do not live in anger but you push down on me harder and harder until you see me react with it. This is not who I am. I dread being in the car with you, at the supermarket, or travelling on holiday in case you can find an opportunity to vent the disease on someone else, to make me feel threatened and flattened. You know this and you must see you are taking life from me each day. I feel no love from you and I need this to fight for you. Your words are harsh. I fall to the words and touch of kindness from someone else because they make me feel good, respected, wanted. You must see what is in front of you — the good as well as the bad. Do not keep pushing away the love that stands at your side.

This latest news is a sickening blow, a reminder to you that no matter how much you try to control others you can't shout everything in life back into line. It is a reminder to me too, of why we came to be. I know now that to have wanted to leave you, to have been so close to doing it, was wrong. My passion to protect you is immense, it just needs to be realised. I am with you, for you, whatever it takes. But you must let me in. You must allow me to help. When it's us, when we are a single unit, there is no stronger match for this opponent. Whatever lies ahead does not matter; this moment is what matters, we can change in this moment.

Why?

John cried a lot in the following weeks, sometimes from the pain but most of all for the people around him. He cried at the realisation that this was not to be an uncomfortable time ahead but a deeply ugly and frightening one. He cried in fear of his children not having a father, in fear of me not having a Lobster, in fear of his friends not having his banter and cheek to enjoy, in fear of his clients not getting the support they deserve. He cried out of exhaustion, to have fought for so long, to have won the fight, to have relaxed and started enjoying life and to have made plans, only to be discarded into the junk pile of reality.

It was about this time that I found a post-it note that John had written on and left in the top drawer of our bureau. It read: Snow Patrol 'Run' (kids and Rose), Pavarotti 'Caruso' (Rose), Pink Floyd 'IF' (friends), Anthony and the Johnsons 'You are my sister' (sisters). I knew straight away what these songs were for. It was sad, it was beautiful, it was perfectly John. I did not believe that the day would come where I would ensure these songs were played at John's funeral. The thought of it stopped me in my tracks, surprised me. This truth did not echo what John played out to family and friends. This was not a sign that he disregarded the cancer, quite the opposite.

John was acknowledging the cancer as a real threat, he was feeling more tired than he ever admitted. I could see it in his eyes, but to an outsider he appeared as strong as an ox with an unshakable will. We both began to question why the cancer had come back. The cancer had not breached the bladder wall; this fact had made us feel safe, we had latched on to it, not daring to leave the confines of its optimism. Why was the cancer there in the first place, why had it reappeared as secondary cancer in the bone? The common causes or risk factors for bladder cancer are smoking and exposure to chemicals at work. John had experienced both.

When he was a mechanic in the army during the late seventies and early eighties they would degrease the workshop floors at the end of each day with an undiluted chemical commonly called trike. Trichloroethylene, its proper name, was reclassified as a category 2 carcinogen – as a chemical that may cause cancer – by the European Union in June 2001. At one point John began looking into research on trike and tried to track down some of his army colleagues to ask if they had suffered any health problems. He did not pursue it for long, realising that it wouldn't change the situation we were now in. It was more helpful to use his energies to focus on what we could affect in the future rather than get lodged in the drain of the past.

John had also smoked cigars, which, like cigarettes, contain carcinogenic – cancer-causing – compounds. John gave up smoking cigars the day he was diagnosed with bladder cancer. He believed strongly that he could not expect the medical world to help him overcome cancer if he was actively doing something that was proven to cause cancer. He would grow furious at seeing patients standing outside chemotherapy wards smoking while still hooked up to their chemo drips. These were not people on their last legs having a final smoke of something they considered one of their life pleasures; these were people with a chance to live longer. We both felt it was a massive insult to the remarkable nurses, doctors and volunteers committed to treating cancer and improving the lives of people with it. After spending time in oncology wards it's difficult to understand why a person would continue to fill their bodies with something they know promotes cancer. These places ring out a brutal wake-up call about doing what you can to protect your cells. Nevertheless, the sad truth is that, although we can offer our cells the best environment, we can't dictate their behaviour.

I found the waiting rooms and wards humbling. My visits made me deeply thankful for what I had and inspired me to see life more simply. On one visit, we sat close to young twins, I guess four or five year olds, and their parents. John was brought to tears; he couldn't understand how children could have this disease. He was in his forties and had lived a full life; these children had been prevented from living, all they had known was drugs, feeling ill and endless hospital visits. During these children's lives, all their parents had known was fighting to keep them alive, not the privilege of planning and hoping for them the things other parents take for granted – holidays, parties, schooling, sports; these were all unattainable dreams.

Another time a man of a similar age to John sat down next to me. We started chatting and he told me he had just been informed he had days to live. He was carrying on as normal, attending appointments, arranging to visit family and friends with the knowledge that he could die at any time in the next few days. He said he couldn't understand it, because he felt so alive. I've heard many people say this: that the cancer never made them feel ill but the treatments did. This man was too late for treatment. Of course we could all leave this life at any minute but when you know for sure you are going to die in the next few hours or days it's an entirely different matter. What do you do? What can you do? Not enough time to experience the really big things you regret not doing, just enough time to see the faces of those you love crumble.

Meeting people like that man made me more aware, less cluttered. I'm not preaching, just saying what these things did to me. I was as guilty as everyone else of living in a bubble. But every time I left the oncology wards I was thankful to be in relatively good health and to realise that this and the freedom it allows us is not guaranteed. At any minute it can be taken away, no matter who you are or how you believe you have lived your life. Some triggers may affect our susceptibility but really cancer does not discriminate; it's in us all, close to us all. Our bodies are full of dedicated soldiers who work to make us function, repair and continue, but accidental opportunity can turn them into rebels. Cancer is one of life's ironic, bitter levellers.

You couldn't make this up

We both had holidays booked for October. John missed his golf, and I missed a trip away with the girls. It mattered not; we were focused on John's operation scheduled for 25 October. Fairly straightforward to replace the hip and the top of the femur. No sweat, we said. John was still physically strong, and everyone around us felt that he would recover quickly from the operation. John's main concern was the impact the new prosthetic would have on his golf swing. Throughout the worsening leg pain, he still made it to golf. As much as I nagged him not to overdo things I was quietly joyful to see him determinedly drag himself off to the course. John never gave in to the cancer; he refused to let it stop him from doing the things he loved. Although to others John looked as if he was easily conquering and dismissing the cancer, I knew how hard he was fighting. Every time I looked into John's eyes I could see his spirit and determination. It is a remarkable beauty that I suppose you only see or feel when you are truly faced with fighting for survival.

Our first meeting with the consultant was far from a success. It remains hard for me to write about it without using expletives. In our journey through the alien workings of the medical world John and I were fortunate enough to deal with well-respected but personable consultants and doctors. I know we were lucky, as I hear stories of cold, self-important gods who roam the wards. Our family practice, John's bladder cancer consultant and our oncologist were a pleasure to deal with, and we appreciated their warmth as well as their expertise. I suppose by the law of averages it was only to be expected that we would spend a torturous few weeks under the care of someone we found impossible to converse with. In hindsight we may have just caught the consultant during an off period, which everyone has. He was stressed, we were vulnerable and in need of encouragement; personalities clashed. It happens. But why at this point in our story I can't fathom.

After a long wait we were greeted, actually not greeted at all, by our consultant. There were students in the room. He gave the clear impression he was running late, did not have time to talk to us and quickly showed he'd not bothered to read John's notes before we were 'invited' into his room. It got worse. We set off down one track talking about the hip replacement and quickly realised that he had no idea about the cancer. When he said it was ridiculous that we were there, that we should have had the relevant X-rays and scans before seeing him, we told him we had and they were probably in the file. The more we stumbled through the meeting and unintentionally highlighted his lack of preparation and frankly rude manner the more awkward it got. I could tell John was upset as he could hardly string a sentence together. Here he was, having had an already long relationship with cancer and about to embark on the next stage. He wanted to hear informed words of insight and support, or at the very least understand what would happen to him next.

I started explaining John's history in an attempt to fill the consultant in on the details but this only irritated him more, to the point that he asked 'and who are you to the patient?' It took me all my strength not to unleash my best eloquent viper tongue and make this ignorant man seem even more of a fool than he already did. It was awful; we both left in a hurry, upset and confused, leaving an angry consultant behind. The last thing we wanted was this man to be operating on John. I didn't want to breathe the same air as him, let alone have him butcher the man I love. Later I calmed down, understood that this man might have the pressure of the world, or at least the hospital, on his shoulders, but I just wished he could realise the pressure we too were under. It was a bad start and I had a feeling it might continue that way. I was not wrong.

It was also the start of my unpleasant realisation that we were now split between the care of two separate hospitals and that there was no bridge between them. I would need to be on the ball and make sure that when we were in one hospital the other one was not kept in the dark, not deliberately – just because of archaic processes, missing paperwork and a silo attitude. At this hospital John was there for mechanical joint stuff, not cancer stuff. But to appreciate a patient's mental wellbeing and ability to recover, I felt the cancer should have been taken more into account. Perhaps it was; we just never saw that.

The hip operation was on Thursday 25 October 2007. We were nervous, mostly because of the impact of the operation and anaesthetic on John's body. An operation in any patient carries risk but the potential impact of anaesthetic, from what I understand due to the way it suppresses the immune system, is of greater concern in patients trying to defend against cancer progression. I sat with John until he was taken into surgery. I felt utterly sick as I waved a goodbye when he was trolleyed out of the ward, facing me, looking more nervous than I'd ever seen him. We did our secret 'I love you' signal and tried to smile over our obvious fear.

I decided not to wait in the hospital; at the time I did not feel at all at ease in hospitals. I was told the operation would last hours and that the staff had my number if anything happened. I came home and sat at the kitchen table watching the minute hand on our clock – the one John had chosen – tick round. I could have spent the time with friends or family but I did not want to be worried about putting on a brave face to alleviate their concern for me. I was also exhausted and did not want to talk about the cancer, or the operation, or the recovery. I was worried enough about the operation let alone how I was going to help John recover while juggling my new job. I'm not sure exactly how long John was in surgery but I think it was three to four hours before I could gulp down the surge of relief that accompanies the words: 'The operation went well, he is in recovery.' Like most other people I had called at the time specified only to hear that he was still in theatre and could I call back in half an hour. I did this twice, and both half hours felt like full hours. As soon as I knew John was in recovery I sent a text to family and friends and jumped in my car to drive to the hospital. I cried for the whole journey. I'm not a great crier; I hold it in mostly and absolutely hate to cry in front of other people. I'm not sure why, it's just I feel I should be a 'coper' and that if I need to cry I should do it in private so as not to burden other people. In the car, where you're in your metal protective bubble, where friends and family can't see you or hear you, it feels safe to cry. As it turned out, the car would be the place I would cry most; on the way home from various appointments and hospitals it would offer me the containment and privacy to let go of what I bottled up day after day. I suppose you're on autopilot focused on the practical matter of driving, therefore the emotion somehow has the space to present itself to you when you can't walk away from it, close a door on it, do a chore to avoid it or have a conversation to dislodge it.

When I got to the ward John was there, still coming to from the anaesthetic. He looked as John always did after any sort of physical trauma – barely alive. His body seemed to go into a deep shutdown while it repaired itself, usually more quickly than an average patient half his age. He was hooked up to a morphine drip that he could boost with a button in his hand but he was not aware enough to do so. He was shaking badly and I knew it was because he was in too much pain. I called for a nurse and explained this was what happened to John when the pain got too much for his body. It turned out the morphine drip was not working properly. After the BCG treatments I hated to leave John alone in a hospital, and incidents like this only fuelled my concern and desire to be at his side watching his every physical response. It wasn't the nurses' fault; they are too few against a never-ending wave of emergencies and demands. I sat with John that night, wiped his face, gave him sips of water and told him that the job was done and now we could focus on his recovery and our lives after that. I thought, believed, we had been through enough, John had proved what a survivor he was. I just wanted him to come home so I could make sure he recovered well and slowed down. I wanted the opportunity to change our focus away from work and stress to health and the people we loved. I wanted John to have the room to breathe out the disease and replace it with life. But I felt a sickening unease that night, though I had no idea why.

I stopped writing this book at the end of the last paragraph. For months I could not go on. Each time I sat down to write about what happened next I couldn't. As I write this, it is over a year since John died and over three years since that hip operation, but my thoughts of this period of our lives, of the cruel twists and turns that ripped through us with no shame, remain deep in me. It makes me unwell to write these next pages, it fills me with overwhelming sadness to think back on the suffering. But I have to write this for me and for John and to show that, no matter how relentless and powerful your opponent's attack is, there remains an even stronger will to survive, to love and to live. When you think it's the end, when you feel deep inside that you can take no more, there still exists the opportunity to experience something beautiful, to find meaning and peace. I don't mean to be poetic about this and I would not for a second attempt to detract from the pain of cancer by prettying it with hearts and flowers. It is a brutal, unforgiving thing; I will not cloud this fact. John and I were fighters but we were also champion cynics, we were surprised to find any beauty in our situation. Yet that is what we gained, while in this stinking swamp, something enlightening and profound.

John was unusually down after the operation and frustrated by the impact of it on him physically. He was glad of the commitment of the hospital physiotherapists who push patients hard after such operations – other patients were not so amenable to this approach – and he was keen to get mobile as soon as he could. By the Sunday he seemed happier in himself as he could see his mobility improving. He was confident of getting home as soon as possible.

On the Monday morning, by simply shifting in the chair at his bedside, John dislocated his new hip. I was sitting at my desk at work and I remember the call, I remember absorbing John's distress, his frustration, his pain. I told colleagues what had happened and drove to the hospital. John was to go in for an emergency operation that afternoon. As we discovered later, it's fairly common for hip dislocations to occur after hip replacement surgery. Well, it may be common for it to happen to a patient once.

I sweated my way through the hours of the second operation praying that another procedure, another anaesthetic would not prove too much for John's tired body. He got through it, of course he did. This was John; no problem our friends said. He was exhausted but relieved that the hospital had been able to operate the same day. So we were a few days behind, deflated by this unexpected event, but we were focused once again on John getting home.

On Thursday of the same week John dislocated his hip again right in front of the physio while he was doing a standard prescribed exercise. This time I did not even switch off my computer as I got up from my desk and I have no idea if I said anything to my colleagues or not. John was sobbing in pain on the other end of my mobile and I was trying to keep him calm until I got to him. He was in anguish, devastated that this could happen to him a second time. Once again he was taken in for an emergency operation that day. The powers that be had decided to change the type of prosthetic to a closed cup. This they assured us was used in younger, active patients and would not dislocate. I agonised again as John went back into the operating theatre for another anaesthetic, another operation. I remember him being wheeled away in his bed and us doing our secret signal again to say 'I love you'. I felt strongly that this might be the last time I'd see John tell me he loved me.

John comfortably ticked another operation off his list and was hugely enthusiastic about his new, improved hip prosthetic. Our friends and family were slightly dumbfounded by the week's events but were not at all surprised by John's resilience. I cried a lot when he came round from that third operation. I really thought he wasn't coming back from it. The first thing John asked me when he came round from the anaesthetic was whether I'd cleared up the leaves. I laughed a lot. Our beautiful home is surrounded by trees, and the weekly clear-ups during autumn are a bind. John hated the place to look at all untidy and he considered leaves on the drive to be as unacceptable as muddy shoes.

John passed the physiotherapist's stair test, a basic check to see whether he was physically able, and got home a few days later. We were well prepared with a variety of gadgets to help John be comfortable around the house: everything from his crutches, to a handy 'grabber' utensil, to seat boosters. We also had our district nurse Claire keeping a close eye on us and especially John. Claire quickly got the measure of John, his cheek and his sometimes dangerous determination to get on with things he possibly shouldn't. I was more than glad to have her keeping an eye on him and keeping golf clubs and ladders out of his reach. By this stage we had become used to pain medications and the benefits and drawbacks of morphine. We listened carefully and paid attention to what did and didn't work for John. I wasn't a fan of the morphine as, while it tackled some of the pain, it appeared to make John paranoid and moody. It was necessary so I dealt with it like I dealt with the challenges posed by John's lack of mobility. In fact, as exhausting as it was, I always considered my position to be a very privileged one.

John hated being reliant on someone else to help him do basic things like washing and dressing. He had never had to ask anyone for help and was desperately upset at his lack of independence after the hip operations. I knew he was hurt and frustrated by the situation he found himself in and I was careful not to make him feel anything other than loved. That isn't to say it was easy. John liked things done his way and there was plenty of infuriating bickering over how I put his socks on, applied new dressings to his wound, cut his hair, cut his toenails, not to mention my attempts at cooking. John loved to cook and was the chef of the house; it was rather a polished pair of shoes I was trying to fill.

My energy was drained from all directions. I was trying to hold down my new role at work, conscious that I had a big distraction in my personal life, one that others might feel could affect my performance. My colleagues were understanding but I couldn't help but see that I'd taken on a demanding job and promised my full commitment at a time when my personal life was playing out like a disaster movie. I didn't want to fail at the job; I was worried that I would need to be the main breadwinner going forward. I had to keep my job, not only for me but for John and the kids, and the pressure was getting to me. I'd be up at an ungodly hour in the morning getting myself ready, then getting John showered and dressed, breakfasted, tableted up and putting lunch in the fridge for him. By the time I got to work I was drained. Then I spent all day worrying about him and phoning to check he was ok. Every night when I got home I felt utter relief that he was perfectly fine and had enjoyed a day of visitors and reading every available news website. John had an impressive aptitude for absorbing and retaining vast amounts of facts and figures and his brain held a fair amount of utterly useless trivia. You were a guaranteed loser if you pitched up against him in a general knowledge quiz. It always made me smile to see this man who had grown up in a council estate in Fife, then disappeared off to train as a mechanic at 16, breeze his way through the questions on *University Challenge*.

John's eclectic, random mix of talents never ceased to amaze me. After John summarised the day's news to me I cooked dinner before we sat down to eat and put the world to rights just like we used to. Then I checked emails and caught up on work often until the early hours of the next day. I never stopped to think it could do me any damage. I was doing what needed to be done.

On Sunday 18 November, a couple of weeks after John got home, we decided to go out for dinner to alleviate John's boredom. We made it early as we had to go to Edinburgh the following morning so that John could get a bone scan. When we could, John and I tried to do normal things that couples do: eat out, see friends, go for trips in the car, go to the cinema. It wasn't always easy, John's mobility was awkward, his leg still sore and for obvious reasons we were both terrified John would dislocate his hip again. We were exceptionally cautious about where we went, where John sat and that no one or thing came near him. That evening we had a pleasant meal, not the best given John's discomfort from sitting through two courses and the lack of Chablis for both of us, but a couple of hours testing the waters of normality to see if we would sink or swim in them. We both slept well that night and felt confident about the day ahead, as if we had left the horrid hip trials behind us and were ready to tackle the next stage of the project. On positive days we approached the cancer like a project, on negative days we tackled it like it was all-out warfare. John looked immaculate, as he did most days, and proud of his improved mobility on the crutches. I knew he was keen to show everyone how well he was doing even after three hip operations. The only thing making him uneasy was an upset stomach the cause of which we were unsure about, possibly the meal the night before, possibly pain meds, possibly nerves.

We got to the hospital in plenty of time and had a cup of tea while we waited. I don't remember why we were in a different part of the hospital from usual but when John said he needed to go to the toilet again I got him to the nearest one I could find and waited outside. The seconds seemed liked minutes as I paced up and down trying to distract my mind from running crisis scenarios. I kept checking my phone but there was no signal. A couple of men entered the toilet and returned, saying nothing to my questioning glances. I knew John was in trouble. I'm unsure how long it was until I heard him scream my name but it was probably around ten minutes. Unbelievably a man came out of the entrance as if nothing was wrong and as he opened the door I could hear John's cries. I barged past the man, swearing in disgust at his lack of assistance, and found John hanging by his arms from the top bar of the door frame of the cubicle he was in.

I knew instantly he'd dislocated again. He did so when he tried to stand up from the toilet seat. He wouldn't call for help at this point because, as he later put it: absolutely no way would he be found on a toilet seat with his trousers and pants round his ankles. How John managed to cope with the next few minutes without passing out defies medical comprehension. He took off his belt and bit into it to help scream out the pain and prevent him shattering his teeth. Somehow he managed to sort his clothing, somehow he launched himself at the bar and grabbed onto it with both arms. So there I found him, hanging by his arms, shirt neatly tucked into perfectly done up trousers, belt fallen at his feet after he called out for help, tears streaming down his face. In immaculate terror I later described it.

Enough of this hip crap; I was burning with protective anger. Whoever the guy was who walked into the toilet as John was hanging there and I was trying to calm him down was very sorry he dared to look as if he was about to take a piss. What the fuck? I knew John would pass out soon if I didn't get him morphine and then he'd fall on the dislocated hip. I ran out to the nearest reception area and spoke calmly but loudly at the completely shocked receptionist. Obviously, even in a hospital, people are not usually found hanging from cubicles in such a mess. She was understandably flustered, as was the woman she appeared with minutes later, who said they couldn't possibly administer morphine. After I dragged them in to see John and explained again that he'd be unconscious in minutes and then they'd face a much bigger problem they began to snap into action. I have no idea how long it was before we got the first of the ambulance crew and the morphine to John but it seemed endless. I talked John through every second, wiped every tear from his face, kissed his forehead, told him what we would do when this was all over and that I would without doubt get him through this madness. I knew I needed to keep him conscious until the morphine took effect and we could figure out a careful way to get him off the bar and on to the stretcher. The ambulance staff were shocked by the situation but as soon as I explained what had happened and what we needed they were amazing.

There was a problem, an added problem that is. The way the entrance and cubicle walls were positioned meant there was no easy way to get the stretcher close to John. We were there for over an hour trying to reassure him we would find a safe way out of this hell. Eventually they got John to drop his arms and weight onto the shoulders of two ambulance men who transferred him to the stretcher without worsening the dislocation. At that point it was the worst hour or so of my life. But I was calm and clear about what needed to happen; I was fighting for John, and the miracle of adrenalin did not fail to serve me. I asked the receptionist to contact John's orthopaedic consultant and tell him we were on our way to the other hospital, that John had dislocated his hip again and needed an operation.

Once we were in the ambulance I felt a small amount of relief that we were heading to the right place but immense anger that John was about to endure operation number four to repair a prosthetic that we were told would not dislocate. How John coped that day, how he managed to get himself onto that bar and not pass out is beyond me. His strength of body and mind was immense. And although later he would laugh with his mates as he told them about getting his belt between his teeth and launching onto the bar, it really was an unbelievable feat. It was not just brave, it was utterly mad. But I understood why: he was a man of dignity and self control, no matter what challenged his reserve.

When we arrived at the hospital I was relieved to see the face of the young doctor who normally assisted John's orthopaedic consultant. He had the cheek to tell me that John could not possibly have dislocated the latest prosthetic. One look at John told him otherwise, though John had to endure the ordeal of a lengthy wait for an X-ray to confirm it. This did not do much to settle my growing disbelief at the cruel and somewhat ludicrous situation which had overtaken us. Then I was sent to wait in the general waiting room – the one I sat in the night John collapsed after the BCG treatment. To my absolute horror they decided that, rather than operate again, they would try to manipulate the hip back in manually. I sat for an unbearably long time, each minute remembering what I'd discovered after the last infuriating wait in this place. Love and protection defeated obedience once again. As I stomped through the ward doors I was told John was in a lot of discomfort and their attempts had been unsuccessful. They tried for a long time and I'm glad I wasn't there to hear the screaming, but I wish I had not seen John immediately after their failed attempts. I thought he would die that day. What had they done to him.

The memory is clear and haunts me still. I thought I would never again see John in such distress. I was wrong, but seeing something worse does not forgive the unfairness of those hours, of a day of events which tore down John's strength not just physically but mentally. Even the strongest of men have a limit and John's was reached when the consultants told him he would need to wait until the Friday before they could operate. He was crushed. He was in agony even with the drugs, his leg was lying disgustingly dislocated and he would have to wait in that paralysed state for four days. To be immobile, helpless, was John's greatest fear. He'd had enough, he wanted to die, he begged for it to stop, he told me he did not want to carry on, for me to make it stop.

Did I want to lose John? No. I have never fought so hard for anyone or anything in my life. But I loved John and I did not want to see him helpless in the hands of inhumanity. This was the first time I really questioned the issue of euthanasia; it was a topic John and I would discuss many times. In such circumstances, those truly out of your control, it's a topic that rears its head ugly or not, spoken or not, as you search for control. When the person you love asks you to let them die what is the right answer? I had to face this question. I had to face seeing the man I would do anything to save suffer in a way we would not allow an animal to. If I am to be joyless, tormented, incapable I would want the choice. Is my fear of loss more important than someone's right to be free? Emotion and fear shade the answers. The question is impossible to answer. You always live with the hope of a better day, a miracle waiting round the next corner. I would not, could not, hear of John giving up at this point. I still firmly believed we could beat this cancer, and more than anything I wanted John to feel independence again, to feel his body and mind on a day that was free of pain and frustration.

It was a gruelling week, where my determination faltered. I tried to comfort John and reassure him that we were waiting for good reason and that they would get it right this time. John was depressed, suicidal, and the morphine was not helping; it was muting his hope, fuelling his paranoia and anger. In truth we were being made to wait for good reason. There were to be two orthopaedic surgeons at the operation and possibly someone from the company who makes the prosthetic. Friday was the first day that it was possible to get these people together. This had to be the last time they operated, there had been enough anaesthetics already and the burden on John's body and immune system was of great concern.

We were both glad to reach the morning of the operation but we were terrified in case there would be an emergency, such as a road accident, that would prevent John's operation from going ahead. As he was wheeled off to the operating theatre and we made our secret 'I love you' signal to each other I was sobbing with relief that it was going ahead but also with distress as to whether John could endure another operation.

I wanted to be on my own again. There were no words that anyone close could give to me that would ease my stress. We needed to get through it, as with the other times, and pray that we would be allowed to recover. Something in both John and me changed on the day of the third dislocation; we were beaten down by it, our hope was eroded, our blinkered eyes opened to the fact that nothing seemed to be working in our favour. We felt alone, no one around us could really understand how we felt, know the private pain and tears. It became easier for me to keep people at a distance during this time; I was genuinely too tired to listen to words of false hope or try to make others feel better about it all. I was also finding it hard to carry John's anger and growing depression. I knew we both needed help from people who could understand our situation but I also knew John would not ask for or accept any. I was drowning in a situation which was desperately out of control but all the while I was making it appear calm on the surface.

Letter to John, Saturday 24 November 2007

I do not normally pray, you know that. I am spiritual not religious. But I have prayed these last weeks. I accept that certain mountains are placed in our paths. If we climb them we are rewarded with the view from the top where the pain easily fades. We remember the growth not the effort, we take from it a valuable lesson. I can't accept that to allow someone to endure the harshest of conditions to reach touching distance of the peak, only to be cast violently to the bottom, time after time, is a lesson in mental evolution. It is despicable. It has lit an anger deep inside me that I did not know existed, it has stolen any bright-side naivete I had. Even I, in my blind positivity, can not justify these dislocations to you. The last, it has to be the last, is the most cruel. I know that lying there trapped in each of those arduous days, hours, minutes has tested you to your limit. I would have done anything to change these days, to take them away from you. I am sorry I could not. We can't excuse this senseless assault so let us not give it the room to scar our resilience. We must protect your body and rebuild your hope. This new anger bubbling up in me is good, it gives me the energy to fight even harder for us. We may have to bend our lives to ensure defences are in place but we will show this shit of a disease that it can not dictate how we feel.

Did John get through operation number four? Yes he did. Yes he did. Yes he did. Unbelievable, inspirational, staggering, bloody beautiful man. There was no way he was going to let his orthopaedic consultant off without seeing his face as we graciously accepted their humble apologies for what we believed would be one straightforward operation morphing into four, each more worrying than the last. On Tuesday 27 November I brought John home and we both gladly waved farewell to the business of hip replacements. I'm trying not to swear my way through much of our story but when it comes to the hip chapter even now I exhale a hearty 'fucking hell'.

It's remarkable to look back on that time knowing that greater hurdles lay ahead in the following months. I don't talk often about what we went through and it's easy to forget just how much we not only survived but stood tall after. At the time you have to cope, there is no option. The survival instincts, the adrenalin, keep you fierce. It's not until later that you realise the enormity of what has fallen upon you. Eventually things changed, we changed, we stopped ignoring the cancer and what it was doing to us. It took a couple of shocks over the course of a year or more for us to reach that stage.

A shock we should have expected

The first shock was the extent of the cancer. What I haven't mentioned in sharing the saga of the hip operations is the other news we received during this period. I don't remember the date we got the news, though I recall surprising detail about the day: the chair I was sitting in when John called me at work, the colour and texture of the walls around me, the muted presence of my colleagues, the background hum of keyboards, phones and chatter, what I was wearing, how I got to the bank machine and then into a taxi to go to the hospital to meet him. I remember John's face, his voice, the waiting room we sat in, Duncan's face as he told us the news. I remember holding John as he cried and cried.

When John called me at work that day I went into shock, only picking up certain words about the cancer being in other places: adrenal glands, lungs, another couple of questionable areas in the bones. The scan results showed a mass of 3.5cm in John's right lung along with smaller nodules in the lungs, which were classed as uncertain. Areas in the adrenal glands, liver and bones were reported as suspicious rather than confirmed but I think we both knew it was the cancer. How had it suddenly gone on the rampage, and why now? I went straight to the hospital to meet John and we waited to hear the news direct from Duncan. When he delivered news to us we believed it, tried to accept it and considered it in the way he advised us to. We trusted him and admired how he chose to treat John. At the time he discussed with lung specialists whether it could now be a lung cancer with metastases to the bones and adrenal glands, a common feature of this type of cancer. However, we later discovered that tissue removed during the hip operations looked like the tissue from the original bladder cancer from 1998. We found it hard to understand as John had been told the bladder was clear and that the cancer had never breached the bladder wall. We also knew cancer moves in the blood and later found out about the immune system theory. It suggests that the immune system can control the original cancer for many years but, as we get older and the body becomes burdened, the immunity subsides and the cancer becomes active again. While this is rare in bladder cancer it's not unheard of, and later tests would point to John's secondary bone and lung cancer coming from the original bladder cancer.

Letter to John

It has increased its assault when you were at your weakest, when your defences were down. It is an evil, cold, ruthless bastard of a disease. A vile, underhand stranger in our home, devoid of compassion, unable to show mercy even in the face of your honour, courage, resilience. It no longer torments us, it is finished with mere threatening play. It is as if the stronger the prey, the more resolute this disease. But we did not invite it into our lives, we do not deserve this, we can close our own front door in its face.

It can march on us physically, it can disrupt our emotional boundaries but it can't take our united soul. It is deserving of recognition now, we can no longer dismiss it but we can protect what it can't touch. It is ignorant in its expectation of total destruction. It has strengthened us, given us the ability to see. A monster that breathes fear into our thoughts, strain into our bodies, but shines light into our being, love into our hearts.

The news made it the darkest of times. Even John's remarkable determination to survive against all the odds could not bring light to those days. He was empty, his will defeated for a time. Although we felt we had already survived an arduous, almost crippling test, we realised we were actually only beginning it. We were exhausted; each time we picked ourselves up to fight on we suffered another stronger, harsher blow. It felt that each blow the cancer unleashed on us was driven harder by its anger at our resilience. The more we fought back the harder the cancer bore down on us. We were on the ground and had no idea how to get back on our feet. But somehow, it's difficult to explain how, we did.

We broke it down into logical parts that we felt were manageable. There was likely to be a course of chemotherapy, possibly a small operation on the lung. On the positive side the bone cancer was not life threatening. While it was unthinkably painful, we'd find a way to cope. We decided that once John had been for the necessary scans we'd deal with one thing at a time; each treatment and operation would be a tick off the list. We were still at this point determined to beat the cancer, which some around us found naïve. We were not naïve. Our belief, our love, our defiance gave us the time we wanted. Yes, John could have given in sooner, could have died earlier, could have saved himself some pain, but he did not want that. John wanted to live as fully as he could for as long as he could. He had things he wanted to do and say and he would not let the cancer stop him from achieving those things. I would stand by his side no matter what, no matter how hard it got, no matter how much the cancer ate away at my own life. My resolve to do this was tested to the limit and became detrimental to me in a way which for a while was dangerous. We should have got help earlier but everything, I believe, happens for a reason. The second shock, the one we needed, came later in our story.

Swinging back to life

John's recovery from hip operation number four was impressive. Really very impressive. He was careful but determined, and once again he surprised those around him with the speed at which he was regaining his physical strength. He did have motivations to spur him on during the first weeks he was home. Firstly he was concerned that his new hip would alter his golf swing. This of course was a priority to John, therefore to me. John contacted our local golf pro Ian who, with similar savvy judgement to district nurse Claire, had John well clocked. He knew John would be more concerned about regaining a good swing than looking after his health so he talked John into taking mini lessons and building up gradually. Thank goodness. By this point I really was starting to feel and look older, a lot older, than my years and was sick with worry that there could be a dislocation number four, operation number five. (Even for the sake of some cliffhanger tension I will not suggest there was.) Besides, to see John so absorbed in golf again and focused on being well enough and able enough to play eighteen holes filled me with happiness. I knew the lows he had reached and I was in awe of his resolve to live fully again. There was one day – snowy, icy – that we exchanged some clipped words when John refused to cancel his lesson. Minutes after he left the house Ian called me and said: 'He's flaming coming isn't he, don't worry, I'll handle this.' John returned home ten minutes later after Ian caught him as he entered the golf course car park and told him that in no circumstances was he attending the lesson, which I should add was to be held in a hut at the bottom of a steep slope covered in snow and ice. Unbelievable.

Slightly, only mildly, less reckless was John's determination that he would make it to his work's Christmas lunch. This filled me with fear. Crowded venue, lots of alcohol, people falling over, icy pavements: again, so many factors conducive to dislocation. Fortunately, thankfully, we got him there and back safely. The lunch was being held in Edinburgh so I booked us in for the night at a hotel nearby; that way John was always close to our room if he got tired or sore. Everyone in the group had my phone number, and John was fairly careful in terms of not consuming his usual levels of alcohol. John was delighted he made it to the lunch, as was everyone there, as usual in awe of the man's sheer stubbornness. I on the other hand was meant to be on a half day to attend a Christmas lunch but didn't escape the office until 7pm. I didn't really care; I was too tired to don some sequins and make polite small talk. I no longer had the energy to pretend all was well; I desperately needed a period of stability, the room to recover myself. Thankfully, we had a quiet and happy Christmas. We were a little stunned and a lot relieved to have made it to the end of an extraordinary year, almost in one piece.

The chemo

We felt ready for what lay ahead in 2008, eighteen weeks of chemotherapy for starters. On 15 January John began the first of his three weekly cycles; he would receive treatment two Tuesdays in a row, then had the third week clear, and so it went on. I spoke to staff at my work who were, once again, thoughtfully accommodating. I altered my diary to be able to ferry John to and from his appointments and work from home on the days John was most likely to feel unwell. By this point my colleagues were used to me dashing off unexpectedly, working from hospital waiting rooms and home and receiving emails from me at the oddest of hours. It was far from ideal and relied on their understanding, but somehow I was making it work; I had to be so focused and organised I just made stuff happen. It was highlighted to me later, and rightly so, that if anything I was working too hard and needed to take my feet off the pedals. Looking back I know I was burning myself out completely trying to look after John and protect my career – our future security. It was madness but I felt I could control work more than John's health so I suppose I overcompensated and overworked myself. It wasn't until my boss's boss advised me that I was giving 120% and should be looking at 80% under the circumstances that I realised they probably thought I was as bloody-minded as John. I was certainly as proud as John and determined to get us through the chemo treatments with as little upset as possible. To date John's treatments had involved operations, immunotherapy and radiotherapy, so we were both new to the process and godforsaken side effects of chemotherapy. We had heard about them of course but until you're in the thick grind of it, and trying to juggle daily life around it, it's hard to comprehend how sodding miserable chemo can be. Necessary, effective, but bloody hard going. Potential results, despicable short-term trauma.

John found the days of chemo treatment arduous, hooked up to a drip, feeling the chemo sting through his veins, in a room full of people feeling equally fed up. I'd try to leave work just after lunch and sit with John during the last hour of his treatment. I knew he hated to be stuck anywhere for any length of time. It was an eye opener and we both left feeling deeply saddened by the reality of cancer. It's unfair on everyone whether young or old. There is a remarkable unspoken solidarity among patients and relatives in the chemo wards; you just have to look at each other to know. I found it heartbreaking each time I was there, and to see older people having to abandon their treatments because they were too sick or weak was soul destroying. As much as you grow to hate chemo you don't want to miss a week of it. You need it, but no way do you want to draw out the agony. Each week you pray the blood counts will be good enough, that you won't catch a bug, that you will be able to sit for hours having this poison pumped through your veins. It is not right. But what is the alternative.

John was given two chemotherapy drugs: gemcitabine and cis-platin. We were given guidelines on how to protect John against infections, as his immunity would be lowered by the drugs, and a list of symptoms to watch for, which we were to record after each treatment. Claire, our district nurse, took John's bloods the day before each treatment to check that his white blood cell count was at the required level. On the day of treatment John was hooked up to the various drips for hours. The machines that are used to control the dose administered make a sharp bleeping sound to alert the nursing staff to change the bags. Several patients in several rooms mean a continuous chorus of bleeping alarms, something that rings in your head for hours afterwards. On a later hospital visit, John said hearing the sound of the chemo machines pulled him back to the slow, heavy nausea of the treatment days. John passed the hours listening to his iPod, reading the paper, doing crosswords and occasionally reading a book, though often he said it required attention he could not muster.

Cisplatin reduces the number of white blood cells making you more prone to infection from around the seventh day after treatment and making you most vulnerable ten to fourteen days after chemo. Your white cells then increase again, you hope in time for your next cycle. As anyone who has had chemo will understand, trying to get family and friends to appreciate this is not always easy. In the end if visitors turned up at the house with the slightest sign of a sniffle I sent them packing. If someone sneezed near me at work or complained of stomach pain I panicked. It sounds obsessive but we were desperate not to prolong the sickness of the chemo or jeopardise its ability to save John's body.

John handled the first few weeks with his usual stoic composure, despite suffering many of the common side effects, such as nausea, mouth ulcers, tiredness, upset stomach and drowsiness. He was glad not to lose his hair: he said he wouldn't have minded being bald but hated the thought of not having his full eyebrows to balance his generous nose. His normally predictable appetite was erratic to say the least. After one treatment he devoured a whole large pizza, portion of wedges and chicken wings, after another he was ready to kill for a hot curry. What he craved one day he couldn't look at the next; he was ravenous one minute and had no appetite the next. It was difficult to satisfy. I spent hours cooking his favourite meals, which more often than not ended up in the bin untouched. Other days I'd make a mad dash to a takeaway to get whatever John urgently craved. He was surprised by how tired he became and was hugely irritated by his changing appetite and recurrent mouth ulcers. But we quickly settled into a routine and got to know which days in the cycle would be bad and which would be better. John planned visitors and golf lessons on the good days and on days he was tired we cosied up to watch movies and endless episodes of *House*. We just went with the ups and downs and didn't stress when plans had to be cancelled or family were annoyed because they had to wait. We had no choice. We talked a lot during this period and were in many ways surprisingly content. I suppose it was more planned and expected than the hip carry-on and so allowed us to maintain some sort of life.

Of course, living on the John and Rose rollercoaster meant that when things seemed almost controlled, perhaps difficult but improving, we were on a steady incline of sorts. We were starting to let our guard down and focus on the view ahead. It's because you relax that the predictable dips still catch you by surprise.

Easter number two

Our descent happened on Easter Monday. Yes, Easter again; it had been Easter weekend a year earlier that John ended up in A&E after his BCG treatments. John was not well on the morning of Monday 24 March 2008; he looked a horrible colour on wakening, and threw up his breakfast. Both of us were due at our respective offices that morning and I had no chance of talking John out of going to his work. John was unfalteringly devoted to his business and clients, even during treatments and holidays, and insisted I deliver him to his work so that he could deal with some paperwork. I also appreciated that times in the finance industry were hard, even harder for small firms like John and Paul's, and that John wanted to work whenever he felt able. The problem was that often he was unable. I knew not to fight about it but I also knew I'd be back that morning to get him.

He called me one hour later to say he was quite unwell, which meant he was most unwell, and that perhaps I should come and get him. On arriving I took one look at his secretary's face, and then John, and piled him into my car. Given past lessons, I knew there was no way I was pitching up at the A&E department to battle through the Easter fall-out again: I didn't want to drive the eighteen miles home to try to get our out-of-hours doctor service; I considered turning up at the oncology wards of the Western but knew they couldn't just admit John without a referral from a doctor and that Duncan and his colleagues would not be in on Easter Monday. The options were limited. So I was a little cheeky and took John somewhere I hoped to find a relevant doctor. Within 15 minutes I was supporting John through the doors of the chemotherapy day-treatment building, explaining that John was mid cycle in his treatment and based on his colour and increasing shakes I expected him to pass out shortly. The doctors seemed not to believe me and were ready to pack us off home until John promptly collapsed at their feet, after which they were all ears. John was in a terrible state and nothing was staying in his body. His skin was burning and he was screaming every time a nurse tried to give him a simple injection. Eventually they got him stable enough to move to one of the oncology wards in the main building, where he stayed for four days in an infection-controlled room. Somehow John had severe gastroenteritis.

At the height of this mayhem I found myself overflowing with excitement as I finally managed to get a hat full of John's poo as a sample for the doctors. It was actually one of those untactile cardboard sick bowls, the feeling of which has the same effect on me as someone drawing their fingernails down a blackboard, but the contents were poo of the rancid plentiful sort. The only way we could find out what was wrong with John was to get a sample, but by this point his body seemed to have expelled all the foreign nastiness it could. So there I sat for hours, with sick bowl in hand, waiting for the goods we needed to get some answers. The male nurse I finally presented it to thought my glee was funny and endearing, saying: 'you really do love this man, don't you'. I realised that yes I did, that I would do anything for him, that nothing stopped my determination to keep him well. And, after all, what was a hat full of crap compared to the shitpile we were digging ourselves out of.

It's easy to be light-hearted about it now but at the time we had no idea what was wrong with John and for the first couple of days he was in a terrible mess, rarely opening his eyes or uttering a word. I was sure he had wandered onto life-threatening turf again. As with the dislocations, John did not remember most of his suffering during those few days. I'm glad of this. It's bad enough that I hold every detail; I'm not sure John would have picked himself up so many times if he had remembered all the physical trauma he was so frequently enduring. Although he missed his next scheduled chemo he was soon back on track, and on Tuesday 29 April he got through his last day of drips and bleeps. We both shed happy tears of relief when I collected him. He had made it. We could focus on recovering into life again.

Positive news from scan results helped to muffle out the bleeping memories. Scans from March, after three cycles, showed that the lung mass had shrunk from 3.5cm to 2.5cm and there were signs of healing in the pelvic area where an abnormal patch had been picked up in an earlier scan. There was no sign of a problem in the liver and, although the adrenal glands were swollen, the view was that it was probably not cancer. The cancer was described as stable. The following scan, done at the beginning of June after six cycles of chemo, showed further shrinkage of the tumour in the lung to 2.1cm and no new disease was seen. It's not enough to say we were overjoyed; I'm crying just thinking about the relief we felt. Yes we were scared too – the shadow of the cancer is always lurking behind any light you find – but to know that all that pain and struggle had been for good reason meant we could accept what we had endured and look forward again.

A good two weeks, a perfect day

With new hope budding in our hearts we flew off to Croatia for a two-week holiday. In some ways it was a brave thing to do but we both needed a break and to touch the edges of enjoyment again. The journey was stressful as John was still on crutches and was weak from his chemo. It infuriates me now when I remember the ridiculously selfish behaviour of fellow travellers and the pointless exercise that is Speedy Boarding. If it wasn't for my manly shoulders and sharp elbow digs to several ignorant passengers John would not have made it to Croatia safely. But we did make it to our lovely hotel not far from Split. I asked for a quiet room at the end of the building, and we got one with a huge balcony over-looking the hotel's marina. I'd been to Croatia as a child, when it was called Yugoslavia, on a sailing trip round the islands of the Dalmatian coast, and never forgot the magical beauty of the place. The genuine people, the almost Scottish landscape, the romantic Venetian buildings, the laid-back sailing communities.

We spent most of the first week just resting, lounging on the balcony, reading, eating, chatting and feeling thankful to be in this place in this moment. We took a day out so I could show John the Diocletian Palace in Split. It was a contented day but I sensed John was a little bored with the place and bothered by the bustling crowds. I was desperate to take John to see some of the Islands where I knew he'd love the scenery, history and tranquillity. There are plenty of organised trips with hoards of tourists piling on and off old converted fishing boats but John was too unsteady on his feet and nervous of eager crowds. I went for a run along the Marina every morning while John slept and one time plucked up the courage to go into the reception and ask how much it would be to take a private trip. I knew there was no way John would agree to spending money on getting him to the islands but I also knew if I could get him there then he'd find the peace and inspi-ration he was looking for. So, after I had recovered from hearing the price of hiring the smallest boat they had on offer, I handed over my credit card and felt sure I would not regret it. Deep in my heart I wondered how many more holidays John and I would be able to take together; travel was becoming increasingly difficult and the stress of it would often negate the benefit of being away. I wanted, I needed, this special trip with John. I knew how impor-tant the memory of it would be.

I made sure John had a few beers with lunch that day before I confessed to booking the boat. He surprised me: no questions or reluctance. We were to meet the boat two mornings later at the marina at an unearthly hour to begin our day's adventure. We were both nervous about John getting on and off the boat and his comfort during the journey but our two sailor guides handled the situation brilliantly. We visited three islands, spending most of the day exploring Hvar's old town with its Gothic Venetian palaces, old boat harbour, enormous piazza and Baroque cathedral. We had a sumptuous seafood lunch and bottle of wine, which we raved about for weeks afterwards, before meeting our two guides back at the boat. When I said how much we enjoyed it but that I would love to have the place to ourselves we were quickly sped round to the opposite side of the island to the most romantic place I have ever spent an afternoon. We were in another harbour with Venetian buildings and wonderful cafes but no tourists, a place we would happily have stayed for ever. We went to Brac for our end-of-day drinks and to soak up the atmosphere of the locals' passion for football as they celebrated a national team victory. The sea was rocky and it was a bumpy two hours back to the hotel but John looked exhilarated, happy and well. I have not had many perfect days in life but that was one of them.

A tough exterior

The two weeks in Croatia could not have been better timed. Each day was calm and special. The memories are precious. It had been a long time since either of us felt peace like we did there, and I'm thankful for every minute. With one exception. John had complained of a niggling pain in his side for a few months and even while he was relaxed on holiday the pain would keep biting at him, at us, a nasty little reminder of things that had been and things that might lie ahead. It would come and go and, while he had mentioned it to each doctor and specialist we saw over the previous weeks, there seemed to be no clear reason for it. We excused it with hopeful reasoning: his limp leading him to compensate and cause back and side pain, or possibly something to do with the chemo. The last two sets of scans and an X-ray in the area showed nothing. To say John had a high pain threshold is a serious under-statement; he rarely complained of anything, from a strain to a destroyed bone, but he kept mentioning this pain more and more. I could see he was struggling with it and it was frustrating that the doctors could not find a reason. This pain in John's side had been our unwelcome companion for a long time by this point; when John strained or stretched, or when he was restless in bed at night, it was this pain that shouted for attention. For now we ignored it.

John was 49 on 6 August 2008. As he acknowledged, he had packed a lot into those 49 years. Apart from our niggling com-panion, the couple of months after Croatia were filled with an enjoyable amount of normal stuff. We decided to keep John's birthday a quiet affair, which was unlike us, and I took him to a great restaurant that we are lucky enough to have on our door-step. I'm not sure why, but I decided to drop off a birthday cake before we arrived and asked the owner to bring it out after our meal. When they did so, with everyone in the restaurant singing Happy Birthday, I expected John to be mortified. I didn't expect to see tears roll down his face. After an awkward few seconds, he quietly explained to me that he'd never received a birthday cake in this way and that it was a wonderful, if slightly embar-rassing, thing I had done. I had no idea, but that was John: a man of many experiences, a survivor against the odds, but untouched by some of the most simple acts of thoughtfulness. He had been a fighter for so long that by 49 he didn't really know how else to be. It took me a long time to coax down the laden barriers and get John to believe that someone could love and care for him unconditionally. It was a rough ride but it was worth it.

John had trouble conveying his emotions most of the time, yet he was one of the most emotional people I've known. While on one hand his rough, tough control would leave me feeling hurt, on the other he would completely flummox me with random acts of heart-warming thoughtfulness. Over the years John infuriated me but he also surprised me: the way he hid cards containing beautiful poems and quotes in my handbag or case; when he secretly topped up a jar of my special moisturiser which I couldn't afford; the time he replaced a favourite vase I had broken – an act he had to draw my attention to after a week of me failing to notice; the hot baths surrounded by lit candles and a glass of wine on the side waiting for me when I returned home after a tiring day; the fantastic meals he cooked; buying a necklace that he remembered me spotting months earlier while passing a shop; my surprise 30th birthday meal and trip away – oh, and the sheep! When we moved to the Borders I was desperate for a dog or a pet of any kind. It was a daft idea as we worked such long hours but I love animals and would not stop talking about it. I also knew John did not want pet hair on his impeccable wardrobe. I suggested a sheep for the garden and joked about it for months until my 30th birthday when I spent the whole day discovering cuddly toy sheep everywhere: in the washing basket, my dressing-gown pocket, the fridge, the garden. If you knew John in all his hard-man glory, these acts would surprise you. He may have had a formidable exterior and harsh tongue on occasion but he did love deeply and truly, especially his children, me and his friends. I always said to him he was like a mongrel I had found at the kennel, a kind of ugly cute brute with a look of endearing mischief but also unnerving devilment – he would be hard work but once he trusted you he would be loyal until the end. Obviously he preferred a James Bond analogy but I never let him away with it.

Impossible to ignore

We were feeling more positive about life that summer and were confident enough to commit to both of us going away for a week, separately. John was excited about heading off on his annual golf outing in November, having missed the one the previous year, while my dear friend Kelly talked me into a week at her family holiday apartment in Portugal in September. I was reluctant to go, anxious about John being on his own. Of course he wasn't on his own but I felt so completely responsible for him by this point that I felt as if I was abandoning him. No one else knew exactly what to watch for, which meds worked and when, who to contact and when. My own health was showing signs of cracking by this point, and John, my family and friends encouraged me to take a week out while things were calm.

John made sure he drove us to the airport in the early hours of the morning. He loved to drive his Saab 95 and had missed being able to during the period of his hip operations. At the airport he insisted on lifting our cases out of the car, and that's when I saw that something was very wrong. I could see the pain he was masking, I could see the upset in his eyes. I was gutted, heartbroken, sick to my stomach with worry and guilt at leaving him. He convinced me he was fine and that there was nothing we could do until his next scan and appointment. I was torn on that week's holiday. I hadn't seen much of my friends for months, and the days or nights out that I did commit to I invariably dropped out of at the last minute. I knew that I should try to feel and act like a 34-year-old but by then my life, and my priorities, had changed too much to reverse out of the space I was now in. I did not want to battle with the doubts or paranoia. I was changing, I saw things more clearly, I was more certain of who I was and how I would be.

I was constantly worried about whether John was ok but I realised that I had to take some enforced rest so that I could tackle what might lie ahead. In the last two years of John's life, possibly longer, I could only really relax when I was with him and knew he was ok. It was often an exhausting pull against my own welfare.

Only a couple of days after we left I knew that John must be in trouble as he called in sick to work and was avoiding my calls. Although he seemed brighter a few days later I felt he was just making an effort to sound that way to appease my concerns.

When we arrived back home, he was waiting for us at the airport holding ridiculous signs as if he was a transfer waiting to collect 'Poo-shoe' and 'Sparkly Princess' (our nicknames, for reasons I'll avoid explaining here). He surprised me again. He looked emotional but was proud and standing tall for me and my friend. John's pride was masking excruciating pain, and it was only a couple of weeks later that we would realise the cause.

If John said he would attend something, whether it was a work appointment, golf game or a social engagement, then he would be there, come rain, shine, hail, gales, new hip or sickness. So, honouring John's mindset, we attended the evening wedding reception of the daughter of our neighbours Bill and Ann on Saturday 27 September. Enough morphine, a stiff drink and sheer determination allowed a man who should have been in a hospital bed to turn up and congratulate the happy couple and their parents. He was in crippling pain but these people mattered to us, and John wanted to shake their hands, wish them well and feel their happiness and hope. We only stayed for a couple of hours, a couple of very stressful hours for me, given the slippy marquee floor and alcohol-fuelled dancing happening all around us. I would be surprised if anyone there saw our fear, our pain. To others we were a couple dealing with cancer, but doing so successfully. When you're not privy to the extent of a problem it's easier to live as if it's not there.

Two days later on Monday 29 September we were given an indecent, sickening blow. We were not expecting good news, we had tensed ourselves to take a hard hit of some sort, but this? The cancer in the bone had spread and it had found its way to John's spine. The disease was attacking the ninth vertebra down. It had eaten away one of the wings of the vertebrae so that it was effectively floating, pressing into the nerves and causing the moving pain in John's back, side and front. I knew that what John was scared of most was losing his mobility and independence, and now this deep fear could become a reality. The news made John increasingly angry; he had fought so hard to maintain his physical resilience against the disease as well as his positive mental attitude. That stuff about being able to overcome anything with positivity and determination was beginning to seem like bullshit to us. We had believed in it, had lived that ethos, no matter what life threw at us. But things just got worse. Our strength had been disregarded, our hope slowly extinguished.

It was perhaps fortunate that an occasion very dear to John's heart was happening only a few days later; it was something to distract him. The ten-year anniversary party of the firm he owned with his business partner Paul was being held in their offices in Edinburgh. There was no way that John would not show at the party, and there was no way he would look anything but confident, strong and positive, which he did with flying colours. Underneath he was terrified in the run-up, worried he would not be able to disguise the pain, or falter and lose his balance in front of the guests, or be sick from all the pain medication he was now taking. He was also nervous in case he had to give a speech of any sort. He had plenty of emotion bottled inside waiting for the opportunity to spill out. Apart from having to carry John back to the hotel at the end of the night with the help of our good friends Gill and Nik – the celebratory drinks had been a powerful combination with the pain meds – the party was a huge success. That night I knew the pain bombarding John's proud frame, I knew the torment harassing his focused mind. But the guests, many of them friends, saw John just as he wanted them to. We were exhausted the next day when we woke hungover and laughing about the night's events, but I was truly happy; John had been able to enjoy an occasion that he had wondered if he would live to experience.

The following Thursday I took John to get radiotherapy on his spine, and a rough weekend followed. As the radiotherapy was focused around the middle of John's spine it affected the underlying systems in that area so John endured more sickness and discomfort. With each treatment I noticed he was becoming more tired and recovering less quickly. He did recover from the radiotherapy just in time for our next hospital appointment, which was for bone and CT scans on 31 October.

The results spat venom in our open wounds. The cancer had flared up in the pubic ramus and the spine. The tumour in the lung had grown back to 3.2cm. I could see that Duncan could not bear to tell us the news; I think it hurt him almost as much as it did us. A person with such a good heart must suffer from delivering news like that to people who are relentlessly trudging through the mire of cancer, one minute hauling themselves forward on moments of hope, the other surrendering to callous retaliations. Many of us have bad days at the office but the work that cancer specialists do, the news they have to deliver to people – some they may have known for a long time – makes you sit up and take notice. It's no wonder it became hard for me to work in the world of finance and fund sales; I lost all respect for what I was doing, how much I was giving of myself to a job which seemed soulless. When you know what a cancer care nurse is paid and what a fund manager is paid it's easy to feel upset by the ridiculous discrepancies that define the workings of our society. Cancer does not discriminate, and when the fund manager ends up in the hospital ward they too feel the imbalances in their harshest light. I saw this once, in a ward of four that John was in: John, a working-class man made good; a homeless man taken off the street to receive his next chemo; a retired middle-class businessman; and a privileged man who had worked at a senior level in finance. All four were dying, all four relying on the remarkable care of cancer specialists and nurses, and on the expensive medications used to control symptoms. I'd been living in a fog of ambition, mortgage payments, bills, children's maintenance money, holidays, long working hours, always aiming for the next material thing. When my sight came back, my priorities changed.

The scan results set deep into John's consciousness. The operations, the chemotherapy, the radiotherapy, all painful in their own right, were not controlling let alone defeating the cancer. John was watching and feeling his body change, and watching the person he loved struggle to maintain work, his care and our home. I was running on nerves and not much else, and it was starting to show. Sleep was out of my grasp, and minor infections were treating my lowered defences like a playground. I was also under pressure to pass my Investment Management Certificate by the end of the year. There was a huge amount of information to retain and my mind was too exhausted to add studying to an already spinning load of stress. John was becoming angry at the number of hours I was spending studying at the weekends, and looking back I can see how untenable the situation was: I was heading for meltdown. I should have told my work to stuff the exam, but I was too frightened about the impact it might have on our future.

We were both worried about John going on his golf holiday to Gran Canaria on 15 November, but now more than ever we wanted him to make it. We knew it could be his last. On the way home after dropping John off at his friend's house I sobbed for hours. Sweet relief to see him laughing with his friends, bitter sadness at the pain he was masking, and overwhelming concern that he would be ok while he was away. I had an exam to sit five days later so while I should have been using the week John was away to try to recharge my batteries I was instead tiring myself further by memorising financial rules and regulations, facts and figures.

John returned from holiday looking as I had come to expect: utterly shattered but as if he'd had a ball. Amazingly he got through several rounds of golf and many more bottles of beer. He had lived every minute with zeal. He was also greatly touched by the support of his friends. In many ways, John was the most physically confident of the group, the one who wasn't afraid of any lout they might encounter. He could handle himself with a quiet and unnerving confidence. As well as having been in the army, the young John had been round many other blocks, as everything from a truck driver to a bouncer to a lumberjack. He was physically and mentally agile, frighteningly streetwise and was usually the one helping other people. On this holiday he had to let the other guys look after him, carry his bags, his clubs, make sure he was ok on stairs and slopes. By giving up his control John realised just how much his friends cared about him and wanted to help him. He was beginning to trust that the people he loved, loved him back and that we were all scared of losing him. He told me later that it made him feel 'happy with his lot in life'. He certainly had his share of life's experiences but the realisation that he could trust in the support of other people made him content.

The bang to our heads we needed

By the time John went for his next dose of radiotherapy, this time on his pelvis area, I knew I had at least passed my exam. It was a relief only because I would not need to find the time to resit; otherwise it felt like an utter waste of hours and days at a time when every moment was precious. By December 2008 I felt like I was battered and bruised emotionally, mentally and physically. I was barely able to haul on my fake composure each day and lock into autopilot. There were hairline cracks all over me. Our first big shock had been the news of the cancer's spread. The second shock came at the end of 2008. It was a car crash.

It was unnecessary, stupid on both our parts, and I was lucky. John was lucky. Although John had shed some tears over the months, I had held most of mine back. As I said, I'm uncomfortable crying in front of others. It's not something I'm proud of but it's hard to change, especially in the company of a man who did not like to see what he viewed as weakness. In truth, John didn't actually see tears as a weakness, he was uncomfortable with them in another person because he did not know how to deal with them. The tears of someone John loved made him angry because he could not 'fix' them and make the person feel better. I saw it in him when his youngest daughter cried – instead of comforting her properly he would often get annoyed; it was his frustration at seeing someone he loved upset. Unfortunately I was unaware that this was behind his anger the night I drove my car into a crash barrier.

We had been sitting at the kitchen table after dinner having one of our chats. The conversation turned to the cancer, to the hip operations, to what lay ahead. I broke down. Not just a few tears; I was sobbing uncontrollably. It was the first and last time John ever saw me so vulnerable. I realise now I should not have broken down in front of John – I needed to be his rock – but he was the only one who fully understood what we were going through; we kept everyone else at arm's length. All I needed him to do was hug me. He did not need to fix anything, how could he? Instead he told me to stop being such a sniffling child. The words hurt me to my core. This was the first time I had ever really shown rawness to John and he responded with such a hurtful comment. All hell broke loose: screaming, swearing, glasses smashed, shoving. We both cracked that night, completely.

I could not take it any more. He would not let us get help, he continued to make me deal with him and the cancer on my own. I don't even remember the comment that prompted me to run out of the house in stocking soles, having drunk a large glass of wine, car keys in hand, in uncontrollable tears, and to drive in terrible winter weather away from a situation that was slowly killing both of us. It was the most stupid thing I have done, and I cringe at plenty of stupid things in my repertoire. I had to get out. To this day I am still ashamed of behaving as I did; getting in a car when I was blinded by emotion was unforgiveably selfish. I may not have cared about myself at that point but I could have hurt someone else. I was in a horribly desperate trance. I gave everything I could to John, and I was worn out. I didn't care whether I lived or died; there was little left of Rose – I was the person fighting for John who had completely forgotten to look after herself. I was lucky that night. I was planning to drive through snow to Edinburgh but only made it as far as the edge of the village before the car skidded on ice and hit a crash barrier. It was a less than aerodynamic four-wheel drive Suzuki Jimny and literally flipped over on its side as soon as I made contact with the metal barrier. That night someone, something, somewhere, kindly tipped over my beloved blue Jimny in enough time to give John and me the shock we needed before anything worse happened.

I still remember the two women who found me that night. I was a crying wreck of a woman trying to clamber out of a toppled-over car, I had no shoes or jacket on and I was inconsolable about what had happened. I was lucky again to have two understanding people find me, not to mention the firemen, policeman and our neighbours, who all dealt with the fallout from our absolute crash. John pitched up at the scene, confident, full of chat for everyone around. I could have thumped him.

I said very little in the days that followed other than to lie to family, friends and colleagues about how I managed to be so stupid as to crash the car in the middle of all our other problems. Most people laughed it off, making a friendly joke of it. They had no way of knowing what was behind it, how bad things had become because we kept everything hidden. We did not acknowledge the real impact of the cancer to anyone, including ourselves. I have never been able to laugh about that night.

Apart from bad whiplash and a large bump to my head, my pride was the thing that had been most hurt – that and a car that was written off. How had I let it get to this stage? How had I let the bubble John and I were hiding in become so full that it finally burst in a way which made me hate myself. But every cloud, no matter how laden, has a silver lining.

John finally said we should get help. He was horrified that he had pushed me to this stage, he saw I was devastated and had fought more for him than for myself. The crash was a distressing way to force us into asking for help but when we did it made a world of difference. If there is one piece of advice I give to other people who are struggling to break free from the grasp of cancer it's to get help where you can. There are amazing organisations, intuitive people out there who genuinely understand, who will help you to lift your feet out of the swamp. It provides critical relief to be able to be completely honest about the sadness, the frustration, the fear you feel with someone who gets it, who does not judge.

Maggie's light

We found our help at Maggie's Centre in Edinburgh. This is a safe place. The building, its energy, its people hug you gently. They really get it, even the thoughts and fears you are scared to voice. They don't judge, they just support you in whatever way you need.

A beautiful lady called Maggie Keswick Jencks is the insight, force and pure sense behind this place. Maggie was a writer, landscape designer and a painter. She showed inspirational strength in living with terminal breast cancer which had spread to her bones, liver and brain. In the late stages of her illness, Maggie shared her energy to write a paper for a medical journal about what she and others felt they needed to help them deal with cancer. 'A View from the Front Line' led to a blueprint for a pioneering centre where under one roof you could find the best way for you personally to live with the disease. Maggie died before the first centre opened in a converted stable block in the grounds of the Western General Hospital in Edinburgh but she had shared the gift that would lead to many more centres across the UK and abroad. Maggie's abundant life-force changed the lives of many. I did not know about Maggie and her family the first day John and I stepped into her Edinburgh Centre but after reading her paper I knew I would write this book. I wish we had gone much earlier than we did.

It was not easy going to Maggie's for the first time. John was uncomfortable, his pride fighting against his need to accept help. He was scared about admitting to the realities of the cancer. He had always remained positive, almost disregarding the cancer as a possible threat to him and those he loved. He was frightened that talking about the cancer somehow confirmed its presence. He avoided talking about his feelings to anyone but me, and he was unsure of the idea of a counsellor. I felt raw and scared that the centre would not be able to help John in a way he felt comfortable with. If we couldn't find help here then I had no idea where to turn next. We both felt vulnerable.

The minute we entered the centre, our defences eased. We felt accepted and safe. We were greeted by one of the friendly volunteer workers, who offered us a seat, a hot drink and a biscuit. Her understanding of our situation was unspoken but felt easily by us. I knew that at some time in the past she had been in our shoes. Already I felt subtly reassured we were in the right place. We were nervous and self-conscious while we waited, feeling as if we had just taken a huge step but not quite sure what was coming next. Even the thought of discussing our story with someone new was daunting. Saying the words out loud, admitting the extent of what we had endured and what we might face, made our fears real and present. Our story was so tragic, tiring and even ludicrous that it sometimes seemed easier to undermine its intensity.

Our first meeting was with Andy, the Head of the Centre. I don't recall the questions he asked but I remember feeling at ease throughout the conversation. John and I naturally and honestly told our story while Andy gently discovered enough about us as a couple and as individuals to decide on the support that would help us most. Of course Andy was skilfully asking the questions he needed to do his job but it never felt like that. We felt as if we were chatting to a trusted friend. At the end of the meeting Andy recommended that John visit him for one-to-one sessions and I visit Elspeth, the clinical psychologist at the centre, for an initial meeting before I joined group sessions. As we left that first day we both felt relief. To be understood, without judgement or pressure, to be supported so intuitively and genuinely, let us breathe again and find the strength to carry on.

By telling our story in a raw open way we acknowledged the magnitude of what we had been through. In doing so we realised our own courage and how strong we were as a couple. Knowing this and that we had Maggie's on our side allowed us to get back on our feet. Instead of cancer ruling our lives it would be a part of our lives that we would work around.

My car accident, the forceful nudge to accept help, proved to be the wake-up call John and I needed to appreciate just how much we were dealing with on a daily basis in practical, emotional and mental ways. We knew we needed to change how we handled things, to slow down, not hide so much from other people, to stop trying to maintain life as it used to be. Our social lives had already changed dramatically but we had to let go of other things too. We stopped having the children to stay overnight so often, and if John really was not well we would postpone seeing family and friends. We both felt it was better for John to see his girls when he was able to sit up and be the dad they knew and loved. They handled the news of the spread of the cancer remarkably well – with their father's intelligence – and I could see every bit of their hearts was filled with hope that their rock of a dad would show the cancer who was boss. I began to stop beating myself up about work, the house, not seeing friends, not exercising enough, all the normal stuff I guess. We realised that we had been so busy trying to hold it all together for everyone else that we forgot about ourselves, that we deserved a relationship that was about more than cancer.

We had a full-blown Christmas with the girls the weekend before the 25th and then spent Christmas in the Peak District with my family. I did not think it would be our last Christmas together but I knew it was special even at the time. We felt exceptionally close to each other and had a lot of fun. In the photos John looks well and relaxed, and when I look back I know neither of us was thinking about the cancer during those few days.

The root of the pain

The beginning of 2009 was about finding ways to control the pain caused by the secondary cancer in John's bones, primarily in his spine. I always presumed that doctors could find a way to treat pain, no matter what is causing it or where it is located. The disturbing truth is that this is not always the case, especially when the pain is in the bones. Regardless of the complexity, volume or strength of the medication, it's difficult for it to penetrate the deep source of the pain. But in January 2009 we believed we would find a way. We began a determined journey of trying everything we could to ease the pain rooted deep in John's bones and even deeper in both our hearts.

A couple of weeks before we had gone to the Peak District, John had a vertebroplasty on his spine. Because of the cancer in the vertebra, the bone had lost its normal density and strength and was collapsing, trapping nerves as it went. By injecting a special cement into the damaged vertebra the neurologists hoped to stabilise the bone and take the pressure off the nerves in the spinal cord. The procedure is quick and John felt benefit from it while we were away over Christmas. But the effects were short-lived and John was back at hospital at the beginning of February to get steroid injections in his spine. Again the benefits did not last. Despite a strong cocktail of Gabapentin and Co-codamol six times a day the pain seared deeply and frequently through John. With each day he grew more anxious, only able to find comfort in limited positions, and our nights were increasingly disturbed.

I have tried many times to articulate how it feels to watch someone you love in unimaginable pain and be unable to stop it. No words fully capture the revulsion of it, the callousness of it: the way it consumes the person it attacks until they are in a semi-conscious battle to crawl out of their own body. Inside the watcher, the lover, the feeling changes from an appalling void of emotional pain into a physical sickness and scrambling desperation for peace to find both of them. I don't mean that sick feeling that sloshes around the pit of your stomach when something bad or worrying happens. It is more than that. Much more to the point, I feel terrified to describe it and reinforce the feeling in any way or recognise the possibility of it happening to anyone at any time. It's difficult to look back without the feeling submerging me; I leave these memories locked away in my outer imagination.

Fortunately I don't remember all of those times. Some of the detail is lost in a fog of holding John while he moaned and screamed and cried, talking gently to him for hours, kissing his forehead, waiting for a break in the darkness where we could find rest. Until the next attack. We did not accept that such pain could be of the human body and out of the reach of modern medication. By February 2009 we were desperate. We had talked about the peace of dying; it was to both of us the only way to escape the disease. John saw no life in this level of pain. I felt no life once I saw such pain was a reality.

On 17 February John found a possible way out. He met with Professor Marie Fallon, Chair of Palliative Care at the Western. Professor Fallon is a beautiful person – incredibly warm, human, aware – who helped us and gave us hope, and showed no arrogance, despite her impressive credentials. She saw all the pain, not just the physical pain. John was alone the first time he met her. He later told me he broke down in tears as he described the previous weeks, months, years. She was in a position to help. With her knowledge she had access to stronger drugs and so John was prescribed the first of many combinations. We were now in a world of serious medications, at levels which surprised us. But the treatment had to match the force of the symptoms.

I would regularly update Professor Fallon as to how things were going. Sometimes I called with encouraging news, other times I pleaded for a change, explaining the pain had subsided for a day or so only to return more angry than before. As with all medications there were side effects. With each tablet another followed to off-set its unsavoury traits. I managed it all on spreadsheets cluttered with tablet names, timescales and side effects. I was tired, and the meds, like John's pain, did not forgive mistakes. I was feeling more responsible for John's life with each passing day.

Around this time I began writing late in the evenings. Not every day, but when John was settled, when I needed to share my thoughts free of a response, question or judgement. For now I tell our story through these extracts. My temptation is of course to soften, elaborate, represent us in the best way. But this is not my desire, and was not John's; we share these words raw and true.

Saturday 7 March 2009

I thought he would die last night. Surely the pain would be too much for his heart. Hours of it, screaming hours. I tried everything. Nothing would help. I begged with God to stop the pain. I made deals with him. Hurt me instead, just stop John's pain. End this please. Make him well or take him but make it stop. This can't be allowed or right or of humanity. I will never see beauty in anything again, you have made my world dark. No strength or insight can be gained from this torture, only destruction. I need it to stop, it's killing us both slowly and deliberately without hesitation.

How did we make it through the hours, each disgusting minute of them? We held on to each other in every way we could and prayed that the relief of the morning would reach us.

He is in hospital now, still in pain but at least he is there and they are trying. He lapsed in and out of consciousness the two days before, not eating, disappearing not just physically. The pain medication has become too much for his system, he was hallucinating, his pulse low. They call it going toxic. So now they are flushing out his body. While they do this and begin new meds his body is unprotected, the pain eager to seize the opportunity. It reminds us that although we might not think that the meds are working, that the pain can never be worse, it can.

I dealt with the doctors and nurses, explained every med, every side effect, the progression of it all. Please help us. I sat with John, talked to him gently for hours, begged him to keep going, to stay with me, reassured him they had a plan. We will get through, we will. My heart, my words held belief strong with my determination to see John stand tall again. My head dismisses the insanity of it all, the defeat that grows within us with each new crisis. I don't sleep any more, haven't for a while. I'm sick a lot, shake all the time. Though I'm always controlled, know exactly what is happening. Constantly on alert to every word, every breath, its next move. I even work, focused and thorough. Too much though, I use it as a counter to the nightmare we are in. Keep working hard, prove yourself, you can handle all of this. You have to. John can't work, he has two children, you have to hold it together to make sure you can support John. He can't be worried about that stuff, not for a minute, so just keep going as hard as you can. The sleep, the sickness means nothing, it will get better, shake it off. You are not the one with cancer for God's sake. If he can fight, you have to fight harder.

Tuesday 17 March 2009

They eased the pain, stopped the trauma. They cleaned him out and established a new cocktail of meds which worked. I spent long, important hours with him, spoon feeding him any food I thought he would like, reading to him from the newspaper, telling him about the world outside, helping him to wash and reply to texts. Despite the surroundings these moments are happy.

John was home for a few days. The joy of bringing him to our place, to where he is happy, overrides some of the bad stuff. We have survived the worst. We were together sitting up in bed, looking at the sun cast mesmerising light across the Pentland Hills, our tears a bow to the grace of a hot air balloon as it drifted up from the neighbouring field and over our place. Our home, filled with safety, with love, each other, made strong by the framing of trees, pretty by a dusting of spring's first colours, enchanted by the birdsong, wondrous as it drowns out the ugly mechanical sounds of our world. We could see beauty again. And so we relaxed a little, enough to find hope.

Hope is what the cancer enjoys devouring. It sinks its talons in, it holds you down. John is back in hospital. But I tasted the hope, I will keep fighting. I want to see John's eyes relax, his face crease with smiles, hear his laughter ring out, have his cheeky comments release my own.

There is a new plan. No amount or combination of pain meds can tackle what is now a collapsing vertebra. We wait for an operation. Another one. It will work. John loves the idea of it. To him it's mechanical logic he can visualise and believe in. On Tuesday 14 April John will be repaired like a car – opened up, jacked up, built up with metal and pins. While they're at it they will cut out the tumours in the right lung. It's not too long to wait, is it. We will be ok.

Thursday 3 April 2009

John has been home since I last wrote. After the doctors flushed out his system he went toxic again, but at least I knew the signs this time. He becomes more out of it, starts shaking and hallucinating. The first time he was trying to assemble something with his hands, mechanical things. He was so determined and concentrated figuring out this drug-induced problem. This time, and it did make me laugh, he was trying to play golf. Lying in bed barely able to move but forcing his arms into position to tee off. He's left his happy spaced-out land of golf and is being fed the latest dangerously delicate cocktail of meds.

It's been ok really. The pain is still there sometimes, jolting us out of rare settled moments. But we are managing. We figured out the routine: the best way I can get John showered and dressed, where he is happiest, most comfy, what he can eat and can't. I'm confident about the meds, what they all do, their side effects and it's now second nature that I notice the slightest change in John: his breathing, skin colour, appetite, mood, the way he moves, what directs the pain's dance from one area to another. I write it all down in case I'm too tired to remember it when we next see the doctors or should we end up rushing back to hospital. The faster I can tell them what's happening the faster they can help.

Why question my role in all this, it's just where I'm meant to be, how I'm meant to be. I'm the person with John, knowing him inside and out, the right one to help him through this. This complete acceptance is easy. I don't have time or space to worry about the decisions I've made, whether this is the path I should be on, what will happen to us and me going forward. My head is focused on surviving each day, one at a time. I care only about making each minute John is here better. I worry not about the past or the future – something that torments my head in times of relative peace.

John and I talk a lot, it's good, really good. The bond between us now is powerful. I learn it's possible to be part of another person. We have to stay impenetrable. We remain sane by resting in a place of deep love, of unity. Strange, in so much pain. And with two such stubborn, independent antagonists normally programmed in fight mode. We are both focused on the operation. We are hopeful. We are scared. Another anaesthetic, a major operation, a weak body.

The tiredness tests me. Sleep, other than lapses into light dozing when John is peaceful during the night, is rare. Work is an utter pile of political, unmeaningful crap. Why do I worry about something that really matters so little? I must somehow be hiding in these mind-numbing targets to get through.

My side really hurts. It was just one of my check-ups at the dermatology clinic. I've had lots of moles removed over the years, they were all fine. My mum's side of the family are the fair skinned freckly lot, my late father's side of the family the dark skinned but moley easy-tanners. I'm a hybrid of both. As a child I turned cookie brown at the sight of sun and as a teenager I searched for the healthy hue on sunbeds, a deadly habit I now know. But my skin and its many little freckles and moles has always been how I am and it doesn't really worry me. But the mole they cut out on my left side has resulted in painful stitches in an awkward place. Every time I lean to pick things up or help John move, the pain catches my breath. I know I ripped them. The doctor said to be careful for a couple days, no lifting heavy things or sport for a while. But what can I do, really it's not important in the grander scheme of things. I had to go supermarket shopping straight from the hospital and I felt something nasty happen when I lifted the bags into the car. Anyway, it will heal. I know John and his shark-bite size gashes heal, so my little cut will do the same.

It will all be fine; if we can get through the operation and the recovery I know it will be ok. I know our families and friends are worried but I know they see our fight too. It's emotional seeing the kids. John doesn't want them seeing him in pain so we need to plan for visits on 'good days' but it's difficult to know when these will be. Their hearts must be torn by the sight of their physically weakening father; the dad not able to fling them about the way he used to, his bravado deflated. I also see the pride and love in their eyes, they feel his strength, know he will not give in.

We are back at the place I have not yet forgiven for all those sickening hip operations, a week today for John's pre-op tests. As eager as we both are for the operation neither of us wants the memories of that place to undermine our resolve.

Friday 10 April (Good Friday) 2009, Easter number three
I should have ended John's life today. Killing the man I respect more than any other, the man I have fought so bloody hard to keep alive would have been the right thing to do. No person, not ever, should feel this. John should not be trapped in this way. I should not be held back, made to watch. Each time we think we have seen the worst it stamps on us again.

Things got bad, really bad at home and John is back in hospital. The pain today was different. Frenzied, frantic, he was clawing to get out of his own body. His mind ripping to pieces as he desperately twisted and turned, stood up, sat down, trying to survive each second of brutality. It was evil, cruelty at its most devastating. It is the worst thing I have seen, I have felt. John begged me to let him die, words heavier than before, his plea pure in heart, certain in mind, felt even in soul.

Now I understand the people who beg for euthanasia to be legalised, I understand why at times the decision should be in your own hands. Yet still it remains impossible: my deep desire for a miracle holding the answer in limbo. Hell is losing John. Hell is seeing him barely alive, yelling to be free. There is no way out of this for me. Either way I shall never forget this, never feel the same about anything again. Life is contorted, out of human touch.

One of the nurses who cares for John was crying. They were not allowed to increase his pain meds any more. The doctors from the palliative care team were reviewing the changing doses every few hours, in between times no one else had the authority to give John extra. I will never forget how I felt today, the faces of the nurses caring for John, the faces of the other patients in his ward. They crumpled in fear and sorrow.

Monday 13 April (Easter Monday) 2009

How do I still function? I live in a repeating nightmare. Why will it not let us wake to light? I hear some of the words from others, they translate to emptiness. I know they want to help, that they genuinely care. They don't know how this feels, I don't want them to. I can't share the truth, it is wrong to air this horror.

A distant place in my mind watches my other life pass by. The family stuff, work stuff, nights out and weekends away. The normal life I'm meant to be attending. Daily worries are barren, common chatter disgusts me. I try to hold on to some of it but it's starting to hurt. When John was in the Western the last time, I stayed at Kelly's flat, just ten minutes from the hospital. She's suffered her own pains in life and she gets me more than most.

We've shared a lot of the good stuff together: honest words, bare tears, lunchtime into nighttime wines, uncontrollable laughter that made our faces hurt. It's good to feel her hug after hours at the hospital, things don't need to be explained or even said. Her birthday was on a Friday and a bunch of our friends were heading to a hotel for a girly weekend. As I could not go I wanted to show her that I still see the world she is in. I found myself heading out from the hospital on the Thursday lunchtime to find a birthday cake and candles, which I hid until the Friday morning. In my ridiculous flannelette bunny pyjamas I secretly lit all the candles and announced my arrival into Kelly's bedroom with an exuberant rendition of Happy Birthday. Is it ludicrous, in the middle of all this mess. But just for those few minutes I felt in a safe place, a familiar, predictable place where people plan celebrations and feel happiness at small gestures. It was my way to dip into the world passing me by, just for a moment, one I will hold dear. But mostly I feel that place, the one where all my friends live, moving further from my grasp. Increasingly I know I may not be able to step back into it. I'm losing a lot of things just now. I know it's the way it is and I know my place is with John but it's hard to watch who I was walk out the door.

John is at the hospital now. Tomorrow is the operation. He is settled, being strong, doesn't remember visiting hell these last days. On this occasion I'm grateful that the drugs numb his mind as well as his body. Though I'm the most alone I have ever been. I'm repeatedly drawn against my will into those images. I can't talk to anyone about how I feel. What can I say, what can they say. At this stage comfort comes from internal reserve, knowing others are praying for you. We got some comfort from the consultant who came to see us this afternoon. He is a calm, personable, confident man with an intuitive bedside manner. It makes a world of difference to be given open care and humour, which John appreciated even in his wreck of a state. John is astounding, he really is. Still able to laugh after everything he has been through, it renews my determination to fight with him and for him.

We feel the consultant will do a good job. John relished his explanation of the procedure: graphic, gory and logical. The adjustable metal cage in place of human bone providing the leverage needed to space the spine as it should be and remove the pressure on John's nerves. The tumour in the right lobe of John's lung, sitting 8cm long and right up alongside the heart wall. They will remove this if all goes well. I pray they can and will. Something magnificent is going to happen tomorrow. It's clever butchery, of course it is, they themselves compare it to Meccano. But there's a chance their expert cutting and carving and sewing will free John from pain.

I say the words, mean them, so many times and I do so again: it will be ok.

Tuesday 14 April 2009

I feel elated. Even now, hours later I'm crying with relief and joy and amazement at the strength of this unbelievable man I fight for. It really is ok.

As usual, I couldn't wait in the hospital. I needed to be at home in a place where I could feel John's presence. Seven hours of torturous waiting, of pacing, of throwing up, of throwing out – half the contents of wardrobes and kitchen – of sheer, pure fear dissolved into unimportance as I hear the words: 'He's in recovery, the operation went well, very well, they did the vertebra and they removed a large section of the right lung', and the 'yes you can visit, of course, my name's Phil and I'm looking after John, I'll see you when you get here.'

I pile my bags together, run out the door, babbling excitedly at the neighbours and drive like a liberated maniac to the hospital to find my John and lovely Phil chatting like they were in the pub. Thank you for this peace. My bloody, stubborn, brute of a Lobster has done it again. My heart is pounding out of my chest with love and pride. I cry with relief. Amazing.

I'm hopeful for the first time in months. We are going to get through this and be able to sit in the garden, cook BBQs, talk into the tranquillity of twilight, watch the bats devour midges with each swoop, trudge round golf courses that would be peaceful without John's endless running commentary, walk lazily in the hills, feel the slow pace of Croatia again, stagger home half-cut from our local restaurant, laugh with the kids, be the old John and Rose with friends and family… dream of the future.

Wednesday 15 April 2009

I felt physically dreadful when I got up this morning. Is this the adrenalin switching off? I feel oddly vulnerable, not emotionally but physically. I took a beta-blocker, was sick. I feel like something is wrong in my body. But I knew I would feel better once I saw John. I did not.

The post-op euphoria is gone. He's in agony. Again. He reached his goal and he's still in so much pain. He only survived the last few days with all our words ringing in his head: 'Just get to Tuesday, to the operation, that's all you need to focus on.' Goal reached, agony remains. It's constructive – not destructive – pain, I tell him. I wanted to slap myself for saying this so I'm sure John would have right hooked me if he could lift his arm. Pain is pain, exhausting. He didn't hear anyway, he looks dead. He lies in intensive care resembling a freakish accident victim with tubes coming out of everywhere. Why did I expect anything else, but we were so focused on the operation as the magic cure, not the trauma it would cause or the recovery we faced.

I want to scream at the doctors. The anaesthetist asks why John isn't taking a particular med – the thoracic doc must know – the junior thoracic doc comes in and says it must have been the anaesthetist team from the evening – nothing to do with her, walks away. Who gives a fuck, just sort it out, put him back on the fucking med and stop avoiding responsibility. He is in agony, not able to tell you. He is crying. Why do they not see the person? Why do they look at me like I'm a piece of shit? I have been handling these meds for weeks, I know his body's signs, I know the med he's meant to be on and I happen to love him, so actually care whether he lives through this butchery we rely so much on. There is a person lying in that bed, a person who has been to hell and back several times, a person we should all see. How dare you ignore him, treat him with such irreverence. I need to see some friendly faces, some people who know us and care about us.

Thursday 16 April 2009

Despite not having the physical strength to sustain it I can't shift this anger inside of me. Anger that John looks helpless, pathetic, ill, dying. Anger that they failed to warn us about the pain involved in the recovery. Anger at the arrogant prick of a doctor who dared to snigger his reply – 'well what do you expect' – when John said he was still in too much pain. The doctor and his repulsively fat ego came swaggering into the ward with his colleagues, more interested in flirting with the nurses than seeing his patients. He does not know John, does not know how brave he was and is, does not know to show respect to a man worth ten of him. He was immature and ignorant and lacking any semblance of awareness. It sickens me. He does not deserve to work alongside the doctors and nurses who carry their positions with honour and care. He is the bad one among the many good ones who make people terrified to go into the health system. I know he will learn one day, learn that his job is so much more than just a job. He has the power to save and destroy people, to make them feel valued or worthless, to give despair or hope. He should respect this power.

I could feel my heart lurch when I walked in and saw John today, despite the nurse warning me he'd had a bad few hours. When a nurse says John's had a 'bad episode' or 'bad morning' or 'bad afternoon', to you and me it means he endured a shocking time. His thin frame is pale, his mouth open, his eyes drooping, tubes everywhere, sweat on his face and head, his hair in need of a cut, nicks on his face from the careless shaving of other people's hands, his odd-looking shaved arms. Not manly, clinical, not right, not John. Like a child, a poor, sickly and helpless child. I'm glad he can't see it and hopeful he'll not remember it. I'm scared I do see it and will remember it. Where has my bold and brash and strong and opinionated man gone. This is a helpless, desperate and vacant body. I said the right things, again tried to talk his mind into seeing the pain as recovery pain not destructive pain. But who am I kidding, he has endured more pain than any living thing should, over and over again.

No one told us about the pain and time of the recovery. Why? And we were naive, we survived so much, the operation seemed like a breeze in comparison to the hell we were in. Why not tell us? We were so focused on Tuesday, not the weeks and months after that. John has no more fight, I have no more to give without destroying myself. I'm tired in a way I did not know was possible. When I eventually leave John after each visit I feel selfish, guilty and helpless. I keep looking back as I leave the ward at his poor, pathetic form hunched in the chair. I wave and he can't see me. I do the secret 'I love you' sign and he can't see me. I'm suffocating, totally suffocating. Make it stop.

I come home, wash down vitamins with wine and write, because the writing doesn't tell me how to feel, to just keep going, to be positive. It doesn't try to answer something that can't be understood or justified or made softer, it is black and white, it is where I am.

Saturday 18 April 2009
I'm on the edge, ready to fall. Tired of the wheel I spin on, of trying to reassure and motivate John, whose emotions and mind are ordered by the drugs not him, of sussing out doctors, of mediating between family members and coping with endless texts. Then the pile of stuff undone and growing bigger by the day: my work, the house and garden, personal paperwork and finances. This and

my own health: no time to exercise or eat, no hope of sleeping. I grow hateful of myself, guilty I'm not holding it all together enough for John. I desperately want to spend time alone, even an hour, with no phone ringing or buzzing, with no worry crushing my skull, no guilt at not being at the hospital or my work. I just want to walk outside, breathe slowly and deeply.

I'm scared at the thought of normal life throwing itself at us as soon as John is out of the hospital. They don't wait, they launch in, expecting to see us, wanting us to deal with other things. Piling on more pressure, not seeing that they are only one of many people adding layer upon layer of their own emotions and needs.

At least John has been moved to his own room and got some sleep last night. Hospital wards are not a place of real recovery. The noises of other patients' sickness, of emergencies, of machines and nurses, slowly scratch away at your mind, provoke your senses until you want to scream out loud to get out. All that stops you is your desire to be better, your respect for the people caring for you. When John can, he retreats to his world of music, lets go of his senses in this world and brings them onto the golf course, to the side of Loch Tay or to sit in the garden.

Today he is angry about how much pain he's in and the levels of meds making him feel so out of it. To lose his physical independence is torture enough; to lose his acute mental awareness is altogether worse. He can't remember the pain before the operation, how desperate he – all of us – became. His anger comes at me. I understand why, I respond with love but it's hard. I'm worn now. He survived a frightening operation, he's progressing well but I know I'll have to wait for him to see this and in the meantime try not to absorb all his frustration. He looks the worst I have ever seen him, like a war victim, shrivelled and gaunt, distant and unfeeling, sucked dry of life. I know it's normal after a big operation for people to feel despair and depression but I'm genuinely scared to leave John alone in case he harms himself. I think if he could take his own life he would.

Today they didn't even help John to get washed. I like to help him to do this anyway: we have our routines, I know the best way to manoeuvre him, how to shave his face and head. But I had a serious financial mess to deal with this morning so I trusted them. I was dealing with cold, necessary paperwork while John was left sitting slumped in a chair. I found him this way when I arrived late afternoon. I walked out to ask the nurses for some things to help get John into the shower and change his dressings; they were stood in a group chatting. Laughing. While he sat helpless, lifeless. I hate them. I hate myself for trusting them. I hate the betrayal of so many things. It's rare to see nurses with any time on their hands but the fact I did at that moment cut me. It's the loss of control, of dignity, that hurts me most to see. John is the proudest man I know. It has taken him a long time, and sheer necessity, to allow me to do the most personal of things for him. I just want them to help him feel dignified again; it can be as simple as him being washed and sitting up when family and friends visit. His eldest daughter wants to visit tomorrow, she's desperate to see him, and she needs to. He is so proud and I'm stuck in the middle. I wish I could protect his children and friends from seeing him so vulnerable, I wish I could protect John from the fear of letting them see him so. I'm exhausted softening the reality for everyone except myself.

Tuesday 28 April 2009

I have not been able to write until now. I'm unsure if it's exhaustion or shock. The hospital let John out on Monday. Not yesterday, I mean Monday 20 April. I couldn't believe it. Yes he passed the 'stair test' but he could hardly string a sentence together, could not wash or feed himself, was still in extreme pain, was hallucinating and suicidal.

I went into my office that Monday morning expecting to work until mid afternoon, go to the hospital to see John, then go to Maggie's Centre at night as I promised myself faithfully I would do. I needed to talk to someone. Then I had my course at Maggie's Centre the next day; again I promised myself I'd go and had taken a day's holiday to cover it. But no, when I phoned on the Monday morning the nurse let me speak to a very doped-up John who delightedly told me: 'They think I'll get out today'.

I was split totally. Happy I could bring him home and have some chance of dragging him out of the drug-induced, frantic, agitated depression he was in but gutted that I didn't feel strong enough to look after him in that state, that I desperately needed to go to Maggie's Centre to recharge myself.

The people at work are wonderfully understanding. Thank God they are. There's only so much pressure a person can sustain. While I hurriedly tried to sort emails and a hand-over of sorts at work John frantically texted: first I was to collect him late pm, then 4pm then 2pm, when on earth was I coming. I could scream and cry, I was trying my best. I knew he was energised to get out of hospital as soon as humanly possible, but give me a break. No one else is turning their life upside down to be with him for hours a day in a stuffy hospital to talk him through the pain. No one else is trying to hold onto their job so we can keep our home and pay for your kids. Then I feel guilt for feeling this way, John can't see the world outside the one he's trapped in. How can he? He is desperate to get home whether I'm able to look after him properly or not, whether it impacts on the one salary we can possibly hang on to or not.

Of course I got there on time. The martyr I am. I should know by now that the discharge from hospital and organising the meds from the pharmacy are always, always, at least 1–2 hours late. I busted a gut to get there on time to find John sat with his bag packed apologising because actually I could have had an extra hour or two in the office, not rushed in the car. Mental note: next time, don't kill yourself, flick the V's at someone and drive through a red light to get here. So I got John home, got him bathed, changed, fed and ready for a peaceful recovery. The next few days were hell.

He spent the Tuesday throwing up, wrenching himself almost unconscious. Vomiting and a fresh thoracic wound don't a happy match make. Back on the anti-sickness pills, calmed, then out of his face again. Apparently because he was in so much pain going into the operation his nerve function is all over the place and his resistance to most meds a lot higher than they would like. Could we have figured this out earlier? Surely someone else has been in a similar situation? Why do we always have to suss everything out the hard way?

Someone had the cheek to ask me the other day: 'So what do you do all day when John's at home?' I never used to believe in sarcasm but recently I find myself increasingly at home in this lower form of humour. I told her: 'Oh you know lazing around the garden, odd spot of housework, make John cups of tea.' Cow. What does she think? Well, there's meds at 8am, 2pm, 5pm, 8pm, 10pm. There's lidocaine patches to change, fentanyl patches to change. I get him up and showered and dressed which in itself takes an hour. I try and coax him into eating breakfast, lunch and dinner, take nutrishake drinks. I wash and dry sweat-soaked beddings and towels so wounds stay clean. I run to the chemist to collect prescriptions, talk to the doctors, answer several texts a day from friends and family asking how he is. I get him a paper when he asks, or a pillow, or extra anti-sickness drugs or loraz-epam – the ones that ease the agitation. Let's just say it passes the day. And yes, I do obsessively check up on him, watch him sleep-ing to check his chest rises and falls and yes I frantically wash the kitchen floor at 8pm every night but it's difficult to take off the nurse's hat when you live with the patient 24/7. There's no night shift to hand over to.

Cooking is again a sensitive subject. It seems that operations as well as the chemo make it impossible to get right. John is the chef of the house, he enjoys it, and it relaxes him. He does everything in a most particular way, his way. God, I miss him cooking. I love to be cooked for. Frankly when we bought the house and inherited a Stanley oil-burning stove I fell in love with our BBQ and our microwave and happily handed over the cooking mantle to John. But John has lost 2.5 stone within a couple of months and I have had to learn how to cook his most favourite meals, his way, not the way of any book or recipe. I'm happy to do so, I'm desperate to help him regain some weight and strength. But he has little appetite and muffled taste buds. His mouth feels burned and from one day to the next he doesn't know what he wants. In truth I spend a large part of my time cooking: wholesome soups, casseroles, bolognese, full roast dinner only to present them to him and have them returned with a third eaten. When you're exhausted it's a little upsetting. Not of course that you let the patient see it. No you must brush off your apron and plan the next meal, hiding the fact you want to tip the plate on his head. I must be a bad person. I'm tired, I'm narky, I would give anything to see him clear his plate just so I know his body has a fighting chance.

So the last few days have been a repeat of the 24/7 caring, cooking, cleaning, secretarial ritual. Apparently the opiate drugs do make patients twitchy especially in their sleep but I've been punched in the head twice and the ribs once, had him try to turn on a cooker with my elbow and tee-off on the 18th hole on my chest. I'm all for such excitement if he were conscious. Thankfully there have been breakthroughs to lighten the load.

For the first time since the end of January I made it to Maggie's Centre last night. How comforting it was to feel their acceptance, to see the warmth and understanding in Andy's face, the kindness and knowing in Elspeth's eyes. Going there is like a huge pat on the back, the type my Grandad would give when he reassured me 'You're ok you know kid, you're doing ok'. I guess Maggie's Centre is the only place I feel normal. The honesty and openness of the other people in the groups is a lifeline for me. They get it, there is no judgement, no empty suggestions, they know what's in my hands. They understand the enormity of what we are dealing with and make me realise that I'm sane and coping ok. Somehow even a couple of hours there make me acknowledge myself, replace the feeling of being overwhelmed with being able to manage again.

Then today John and I went to see Professor Fallon. I was so relieved to see her and hear her talk to us warmly and eloquently about John's post-op pain triggers, behaviours and responses to drugs. I'm in awe of the way she holds such knowledge and influence but doesn't lose herself in it – she is always fully aware of John as a person not just as a drug recipient. The upshot is that John is still in a lot of pain but it shows all the signs of nerve pain from where they 'jacked open' his ribs to do the operation. This means (a) it's normal and (b) it's treatable. Wonderful. A straightforward problem, prognosis and answer – not something we usually specialise in.

Then we saw our other favourite medical friend, our oncologist Duncan, who chatted through the post-op news. The hospital analysed the tumour removed during the operation and it does seem to show the characteristics of bladder cancer, which has progressed to the lungs and then the bones. The good news is that bladder cancer is a comparatively friendlier beast. They also confirmed they removed all the cancer from the lungs.

So today, Tuesday 28 April 2009, is sort of a good, encouraging at least, day. Relatively speaking of course. John is still out of his face on drugs and shouting in pain every time he moves. I'm throwing up, when it's convenient, and shaking a lot. And I botched tea again. None of that matters tonight, what does matter is that we both feel hope. Again.

Tuesday 2 June 2009

It's a month since I last sought refuge in the keyboard. That hopeful feeling of 28 April allowed John to recover gently, to eat better, to come back into being John again. We talked a lot and cuddled in the only pillow-supported, contorted ways that allow it to be comfortable. We spent valuable time with the kids and friends. We soothed ourselves in moments of ease and contentment. There have been a couple of surprises. Not disastrous, not pleasant either. The thing about having, rather than choosing, to live in the moment is that you don't spot the stuff approaching even though it's been visible in the distance for a while.

First was the money thing. John works in financial services, not an easy world to operate in during credit-crunch time. Things have been getting steadily tougher. We haven't been able to deal with it, Paul has been kindly trying to protect us from it. But the hard truth is that John being unable to bring in clients is crippling an already stressed business. We need to face up to it and sell the house, the home John loves. We overextended ourselves getting it and now there's no safety net. I feel even more pressure to work hard at my own career; we will rely on it now more than ever. It terrifies me, the thought of losing my financial security. I went through all that as a child, lost my home, lived in emergency accommodation. It's what drives me so hard – not wanting to go back to that. John is similar, though for more complicated reasons. He always says he doesn't have future aspirations as such but that he knows he does not want to go back to the life he was raised in. Any chance of sleep is out of the window; my adrenalin whitewashes my ability to rest. I'm popping beta-blockers and sleeping pills to no obvious effect. But I am in control, the estate agents and surveyor have been round, the place was pristine, the photos for the schedule look great. John is devastated. He does not want to be anywhere else but here. If he's going to have limited time he wants it to be here. If there is a way I will make this happen.

Second was the call from the hospital. About me, not John. 'The mole you had removed from your left side, we were right to do so.' I'm not sure what was said next except the words malignant melanoma and wide excision. I was at my desk at work when I took the call and just remember thinking that I am the carer, I can't possibly have cancer, it's definitely not possible. I cried but I don't know why as I felt nothing. I had to call John, who sounded worried sick – the hospital had called the house first asking to talk to me but wouldn't say what about. I have never, even through all the unfairness dealt to him, heard John sound so sad and worried.

I went to the hospital a week later to get a wide excision. They cut out a larger area around where the cancer was detected. The bad news is that if you're going to get skin cancer this is not the one to get. Good news is it's a thin melanoma. My mind: I'm covered in moles and freckles how on earth do I keep an eye on all these, I know what this cancer does to people, I see it. Why this cancer? Why not one I know how to deal with. I have been so stupid; if John had not noticed the change in this small mole I never would have gone to see about it. This is my fault entirely and now it will interfere with me looking after John. It must be there to tell me something. Is it reminding me to feel for me not just for John? Their words ring in my ears: 'probably a very good prognosis though we can never say never with melanoma'. Round and round and round.

The mess of my stitches from when the mole was removed did not impress the doctor. When I explained why I couldn't really adhere to the guidance notes about protecting them he decided that he would follow the wide excision with double stitching: dissolvable stitches plus a running one. It hurt. In the week that followed I boasted a raging cold, urine or kidney infection and a bitch of a time at work. What a mess. But is there an ironic answer staring straight at us? I started to look at my critical illness insurance, my grumpy little mole may be the way to ensure John is where he wants to be.

John's been on much better form, sitting in the sun memorising the papers, that annoying but impressive thing he can just do. I detect this positive face is for me rather than a true reflection of his biological wellbeing. There's a new pain, on the opposite side to where the op was done. He's angry and frustrated when he feels it pester him. The pain team have brought forward his scan and upped his meds.

The weird thing is that because so many aspects of our life appear to be on a trajectory straight into the reeking heart of the shit heap there's no point worrying. We've lost control completely so what can we do? In isolation the individual events seem overwhelming, like each is the end of the world. But with most of our worst fears all siding up to us at once, forming an impenetrable cage around us, somehow their individual force is diluted. I think we are at the point of not caring. I challenge you to keep throwing knives at us, go on, do your worst, you can't hurt us anymore. It must be how people survive the horrors of war, initially with adrenalin and then in numb shock.

We have laughed a lot in the last few days. If our story is to allow this incongruous disease to take us both before our time then let's disappear on an extended holiday blast and then check in to Dignitas. There is meaning in this proposal. For now we are home, eating my less than perfect food, popping our pills, drinking Chablis with *House* and Jack Bauer and casually smelling sweet roses in the heart of our shit heap. In this moment I feel that together, whether it's drug induced, shock induced, nothing-to-lose induced, we are happy. Us, the only certain thing right now, is good.

Friday 3 July 2009

I missed a month again. Not sure I can form thoughts any more, let alone words on a screen. There were more scans, more radiotherapy. That niggling pain was trying to tell us something. Duncan scheduled us in for five lots of radiotherapy to various areas: left ribs, a vertebra two down from the one replaced, left side of his pelvis, another vertebra even lower down, and his right knee. Fucking cancer.

On Tuesday I took John to the Western for a radiotherapy session at lunchtime. First we had an appointment with Professor

Fallon. John is weaker by the day, often he seems barely conscious. But I helped him get up, washed and dressed – he would only present himself smartly to Professor Fallon and Duncan – and drove to the hospital. It was a long journey, John was moaning in pain and I had to stop twice to give him extra pain meds. We had to get there, we couldn't miss any chance to alleviate John's pain. He was so ill in Professor Fallon's office she let him lie down on her treatment table to rest until we could go to Radiology. I could see a change in her eyes, not one I liked.

Today is hot, clammy and thundery here. Too hot to be dealing with sickness, work emails, cleaning bedding and running up and down flights of stairs. Upstairs John is living, surviving, but he looks to anyone else like he is dying. Downstairs I hear bizarre background commentary to this nightmare. The washing machine is grumbling ferociously – don't dare give up on me just now – the hypnotic noise of a tennis ball being whacked back and forth to the cheers of fans is now over, Andy Murray has just been knocked out of the Wimbledon semi-final by Andy Roddick. I can feel the nation sigh. Now I hear the murmuring of post-match analysis, it's annoying me but I need to lie down. This is more than tiredness.

When we heard about the cancer spreading to other vertebrae our immediate fear was for another operation. Neither of us are ready for that, now, if ever. I was relieved to hear they caught it soon enough that radiotherapy should work. I'm now scared that John is too sick from all the meds to cope with the radiotherapy. But he needs the radiotherapy to lessen the pain so they can lessen the meds. Where are we going from here? I've been on the phone to the doctors a lot, getting advice about how to tweak each med I'm giving to John. It's a fine balancing act, one tablet offsetting the effects of another, nothing quite the right measure yet.

Claire is here a lot, thank God. Our district nurse is as sharp as John and as dedicated to his care as I am. From the first time she met John, way back at hip replacement number one, she sussed his stubbornness, pride and complete disregard for any feelings of illness – minor or life threatening. Since then she has got to know us well, warts and all. She keeps us on the right track without us even knowing it. We trust her judgement and value her support. If I could not call upon her and our local doctors I would maintain only half the strength I do. Maybe I'll feel better when she arrives, maybe John will be better by then.

Wednesday 8 July 2009
Really I'm far too tired to write tonight but I know this day is significant and that at a later date I will need these words to figure out what happened. I had two hours sleep last night followed by a long, traumatic day. No one, not I, not Claire, not the doctors here or at the hospital, not pain specialists can find a way to stop John being sick. He hasn't eaten in days. He can't hold down fluids. He's had various anti-sickness drugs but his body rejects even the lifeline of small drops of water. The sickness is relentless. Watching John's weakened frame violently retching is torturing me. I beg it to stop, I beg John to hold faith, to stay with me.

At some point one of the doctors mentioned doing a brain scan; it would explain the sickness. I am scared. More than ever before. I am not ready for this. Then one of our own doctors called me. They have to get John into hospital before the weekend. The oncology wards at the Western are full. We could look at admitting John to a Marie Curie hospice not far away; how did I feel about this? In the seconds I stopped to think I wondered, despite her reassurance otherwise, if this was their way of getting John and me to step into the next stage. I knew that people went to a hospice for pain relief and day stays, that it was much more than a place to die, but it had not been mentioned before.

There was no time to think about it. The local doctors would be closed over the weekend, it would be different on-call nurses from further away. I had to make sure a doctor was monitoring John continuously; we had to stop him being sick; we had to get him stable and sort out these meds once and for all. So, not for the first time, an ambulance was called to the house. I knew what to do, what to give to them. I knew what to say to John to keep him calm. I knew to bundle all his meds, together with my spreadsheet with every detail I could possibly need to pass to a new doctor, into John's hospital bag. I knew to take my own car instead of going in the ambulance to avoid hassles with transport later. I cried the whole way there. It felt different this time.

I remember the faces of the nurses when we arrived. Their baffled eyes watching this woman with her spreadsheet and meds and concise, accurate summary of exactly what had happened and the key things to look for in John in terms of reactions to pain and meds. It struck me that I looked more at home in this world than in my own.

I know we're in the right place, a good safe place. The nurses and doctors I spoke to understand the state John is in, they have the means to make it easier. They reassure with talk of flushing out John's system and implementing a new med regime with drugs more likely to get to the root of the pain, drugs that can only be administered to John in the hospice, drugs too strong for our local doctor to prescribe, too dangerous for me to be monitoring. It does not feel like a hospital, the energy in the place is surprisingly light and restful. I think it's from the people. I know that when John is able to open his eyes and sit up he will be relieved not to be in a hospital ward. He will look out of the large windows of his own room to the rolling view: the opposite side to the Pentland hills that we look out at through our bedroom window. He is settling already. It is going to be ok.

Thursday 9 July 2009
Professor Fallon called me this morning. She said she was returning a call I made to her previously. Really she called to make me accept. It is fair of her to do so, it is kind. I have to hear the words when they come from her. She knows the truth and she knows we are blind to it. I hear these words but they must be from someone

else's story. These words do not match John and me; these words must not take hold, must not matter, only what we feel is real. We can change words, ignore them, make our own. John will not accept it. I am not ready to. Not this fast. We've stood up again and again, we can't fall for the last time.

I can't breathe. Something is exploding in my heart. My skin is burning. I know I am crouched on the carpet being sick but I do not feel anything under me. My body holds no weight, my mind is pulling backwards out of my head. The walls are moving out into nothingness. I see myself on a torn piece of rug, everything around it shattering into pieces, drifting away from me. I am falling fast. There is no way to stop it.

Thursday 16 July 2009

It's a week since I was told John had days to live.

I had to tell John. I had to believe the words enough myself to make John accept the reality. He did not. John does not feel 'dying'. He will live each breath until he dies and in the meantime he has no interest in the business of dying. There is life and death, no in between.

He looked at me as if I was betraying him – us – by saying the words I'd been given. As if he was trying to make sense of some ludicrous suggestion. It did not help that his mind was numb from the new drugs; I would need to talk to him again when he was more lucid. How cruel that I had to deliver these words, which had already stolen a part of me, for a second time.

When I could see John, my Lobster, looking back at me free of the medicinal haze I told him again. It made no difference. He owns each breath no matter how laboured it may be. I feel the same. I am not ready for this to be the end. I do not believe these words, so how can he.

In the days that followed we held each other, talked a lot and listened to the beautiful people who work in the hospice. In our time alone we laugh and love truly in moments sacred, everlasting.

We are free of concern for daily life, of the past and the future. We are shipwrecked on an island, we can see our belongings, our obligations bobbing in the waves, drifting further out each day, the noise of the mainland, of everyone around us becomes more distant. We are bare, totally bare and basking in the light of peace.

We accept that John's body can no longer defeat the cancer, that he is, in their words, terminal. We do not accept a time-scale of days or weeks. There are things still to say, still to do. John, I know, will not set his soul free until he has done these things. Whatever this means I will help him. We need more time and we will take it. John is 50 on 6th August. He laughs at the suggestion that he is unlikely to see this day. There is no way he is not making it to 50. I know without hesitation, without doubt, that he will be with me on that day. So now we are in a new rou-tine to get us there, regardless of what anyone else may believe.

There has been a lot of emotional pain, that of his children, his friends, his sisters. John is settled in his own knowing, watch-ing the people in his life move around him and engage him, share the words gone unsaid for too long. There is no time for pettiness now, no time to listen to those who can't let go of it. There are those whose aim is to be free of their own guilt before John dies, and we see it. John can take stock, can see the colours of each person around him. His children and his friends light him up and he loves it. He's here for them and for me. His need to tell us is more important than manly composure. He's easy with who he has been and who he is. John will make sure he has organised what he needs to and that the people he loves and respect know it.

My mind is free; it's my body that reminds me of the world outside. My joints and muscles ache, my neck and head hot from searing pain, my stomach rejects food and the pills that stop my heart thudding. Emotionally I'm numb, living for John, happy not to think of what this means for me. I yearn for the moments on our island. When we are not there the noise of it all is suffocat-ing. Text messages, phone calls, doctors, nurses, visitors, more and more questions. We are desperate to be alone and peaceful without the warring thoughts of others, their guilt, frantic attention, without the ignorance of people in the practical world, in the companies that you have to speak to at a time like this.

But I'm glad that John and I and these guardians from the hospice are all working to get John home. Now they know us, they see John will not accept the end until he has his time at home and they believe in us getting it. The nurses are going to train me up on how to give John some of his meds before he is allowed to come home. They trust me to do it. This responsibility makes me realise how dangerously tired I am. I must try to get some sleep while I can so I can concentrate when he comes home. It's distressing to leave him at night, hard not to stay awake in case the phone rings. Tomorrow I accompany John to the Western for a head scan at 9am. I will not be gifted sleep tonight no matter how many pills I take.

Saturday 18 July 2009

We got to the Western; it was difficult but we got there. The cancer is not in John's brain. John and our friends who know us well enough to cross the lines of politeness joked that there is no brain there to attack, though we all know it's some of the sharpest matter around and we would all hesitate to challenge it. If only the relief and laughter would endure. The disease stays where it has gained an advantage, the bones. Here it will destroy more slowly, more painfully. Where it already was it has grown and in new places it settles in with force.

The day has been too long, all about pain. Each time he is restful I lapse into a false sense of security only to be hauled out of it by the speed and intensity of the latest onslaught of agony. My attempts at settling him, talking him through it, giving him every bit of energy I have, steadily take their toll. In some moments I feel I'm losing him, he closes to life outside him and the hospice, he withdraws seamlessly from present, from memory, from reality. Meanwhile I fall out of control into reality.

Tuesday 21 July 2009

I'm scrambling my way through this now. I had no idea what true exhaustion was, its crippling force when it engulfs you. I need air. I need life. My body is fighting harder than ever and will not allow sleep, no matter what.

I get up, throw up, prepare a new bundle of clean clothes for John, drive to Edinburgh, stop for John's favourite coffee at a kiosk in Morningside, get whatever food he fancies from the Marks and Spencers next to it, chat to John while he drinks his coffee and eats his croissant, get an update from the nurse on duty overnight, buzz for extra pain relief, help John get showered and dressed, put dirty washing to one side, wait for doctors coming round, help John with lunch, let him sleep, answer texts, co-ordinate visiting times with everyone, talk to John, see another doctor, nurse, buzz for extra pain relief, help John to the toilet, buzz for extra pain relief, help John with tea, welcome visitors, say goodnight to John, cry my way home in the car, deal with all the phone calls, reply to all the texts, open mail, worry, write down a list of things John will want to know, put on washing, go to bed, lie awake. Repeat. Surely each minute should be consumed with John and me, not empty practicalities.

My relief, my support, my foundation come from the nurses. They understand, they see, they give the help we need, they make it easy to trust them. I know all of them on John's floor now and they feel like family. I know I must be careful of depending on them, but they are there with John and me at our most vulnerable, sharing our tears and our laughter. I feel humble in their presence; this is not an occupation, a job they do. It is vital.

Carmen with her keen eye and adorable manner is teaching me to do the breakthrough meds. John's core combination of drugs is supplied via a syringe driver; when John comes home our district nurse will change this critical supply every 24 hours. The breakthrough meds are the extra painkiller 'shots' I can give John as he needs them, most likely before/after physical movement like washing or moving any distance. I know that along the way I have built up reliable knowledge of all the oral meds, their combinations and side effects, but injecting the alfentanil and diamorphine into John is new to me and frightening. I know I will have Claire there each day, changing the syringe driver and checking on us morning and afternoon, I know I have many people at the end of the phone, minutes away, but sometimes it will be just John and me. I don't want John's life in my hands but I realise it has been this way before now. Somehow my adrenalin keeps me sharp despite the missing sleep, and deep down I know that no one will give themselves so completely to John's care as I do. We are meant to be together in this moment, of this I have no doubt. We are meant to find each other, ourselves and peace in this moment.

I went to see Andy at Maggie's Centre today. I realise that I'm so focused on what life looks like that I have no idea what death will look like when it begins to arrive. I'm terrified of how I will be without John but I'm not scared of the actual act of dying. John is not either. We both joke that it's living that's the scary bit. John says he's here or he's not. When he's not he won't be worrying. But while he is here he's worried about what I face after he goes. John has been in so many states of semi-consciousness, looked like he was dying so many times, only to look bright as a button days later. How can I be sure when it's his time?

He defies the doctors' conventions. They say he should not be able to endure so well the cancer or the level of drugs he is on, that he should feel so much more unwell. One of the senior doctors tells me he has never met anyone like John that it seems his brain does not register feeling unwell. John will say he's in pain but he never responds that he feels unwell. They have warned that because John is such an 'unknown', responding in unexpected ways, he could die very suddenly or take much longer. I know in my heart that John will be here until he has done what he wants and needs to, and when he makes his mind up to let go he will die peacefully and suddenly. No grey area. Here in full, then not at all. That is what I feel. I hope it is right.

I can ask questions at Maggie's Centre which I don't feel comfortable asking anywhere else. How will John actually die? What will cause it? How long will it take? How will he look, feel, be? How do I know when it's going to happen? My greatest fear is not to be with John when he dies. But I need to be away from the hospice sometimes to do things for John and prepare for him coming home. It could go on for days, it could go on for months. By the time I left Andy I felt more informed about the different circumstances I might face. To help John I must not show alarm or fear, I must be calm. Uncertainty is often the greatest weight to carry, and John and I have always felt better asking questions to get honest answers, reading what we need to. I've read the honest information from the hospice on dying, the signs to look for. I have done all I can to prepare. When I know John is ready to go I must let him do so; I know he will not leave until he knows I am ok. This will be the hardest part. Loving and trusting to the point I can let him go. This no one can prepare me for.

I stayed late at the hospice tonight. We were enjoying our time together talking about what we would do when John got home. He wants peace and time to just be. He wants to see his friends and kids. He wants to sit at his desk, read the paper from cover to cover and sit back, gaze out of the window at the trees and feel his home around him. He wants to see colour in the garden and soak in life. He wants us to be together content: curled in next to each other without a word spoken or sitting for hours talking about everything and anything until we succumb to sleep out of necessity. I feel we will have those things but part of me fears that each time I say goodbye it will be the last. I remember the last time I hugged my granddad. He was perfectly well that day but I knew it would be the last time, the strength I felt from him, the unspoken words, the unconditional love from each one of us to the other. I cried all the way home from Tayport to Edinburgh knowing that the rock of our family would not always be there. So I should know with John, I must do.

Before I left John, we stared out of the windows awestruck by the view. It was hard to believe it was real. A patchwork of different weather playing out for miles upon miles across the untouchable sky, the Pentland Hills lapping up rain and hail from skies blue, grey, clouded and clear, at the heart a glorious ribbon of colour from the most vibrant rainbow I have seen. We felt lucky. I said goodbye to John in uninterrupted sunshine.

Ten minutes later I was driving through the heart of a ferocious storm. Lights at full, hands tight on the steering wheel, eyes peering to see, I felt my luck fall away under the wheels. I see the storm on my horizon. I have only fate at my side.

Saturday 25 July 2009

What a bloody beautiful day. We did it. We were allowed home for the day as a test run. I thought I would explode with frustration this morning as we waited to get all the checks done and the meds prepared, worried John would take a turn for the worse before we were allowed to leave. Packed to the gunnels with meds that would make a dealer blush we tentatively got home to the welcome of a glorious summer's day. I shall never forget John's face as I got him out of the car to walk into his home; he cried with relief.

The journey was difficult. John was overcome at being exposed to the joys of normal life: people out walking their dogs, cycling, shopping and golfing. I felt his pain at seeing what was now out of his reach. Once he was home he forgot, he was safe and happy. I was nervous about the meds but we got through it. Looking at him settled in his chair in the sun reading the paper, the cancer was nowhere to be seen. I'm grateful for every single moment of this sunny day. I wish I had not taken the sunny days of our past for granted.

We had tea on the decking and shed tears when it came time

to take John back to the hospice. It was a day we both wanted to live in forever. We were excited to tell the nurses how well it had gone, though our beaming faces negated the need for words. I stayed for a while then returned home to get everything organised for tomorrow. Once we see the doctor on morning rounds, I can bring John home. I'm overjoyed.

Sunday 26 July 2009

It's not fair. No one deserves this. Why do this to us? Why pick us up only to throw us back down again?

John called just after 8am, his voice overcome with upset and fear. John does not get scared. He can't move his legs. I died inside. Today was our day, the first of many; do not take it away.

There are no words for today. It sickens me. The doctors and nurses showed hurt for us as they tried to explain that one of the tumours is putting pressure on John's spinal cord. We need to go back to the Western for intensive radiotherapy. The news crushed John's spirits. He could feel the comfort of being home only yesterday and now he faces going back to a ward. His hope has left him today. He is retreating to a place deep inside where I'm struggling to reach him. Please make this for a reason, please let him come home to me.

Wednesday 29 July 2009

The first day of radiotherapy. The cancer has grown but not where we thought. It's where John had the vertebra replaced. After that brutal operation, how dare this disease take hold there. The butchery, the exhausting recovery for no reason at all. It just keeps gnawing at us, letting us loose to run for short periods before it drags us back to the ground attacking open wounds and ripping open new ones. It's resurrecting in the lungs, and the adrenal glands are now definitely diseased.

At least in nature the kill is for a reason and it's usually fast. There is no sense, no need for this.

A tumour is pressing into John's spinal cord interfering with his ability to walk. There are spots of it all over his spine. I'm deeply thankful that the hospice recognised what was happening straight away. They pumped John full of steroids to reduce the swelling and pressure on the spinal cord. This means we have a chance of getting John back on his feet. I pray that he can move his legs and walk. I would give anything to prevent John from being paralysed. He can not end his life feeling helpless.

I go to bed glad this happened in the hospice before John came home. We would not have been able to react so quickly at home. The hospice may have saved his movement and dignity, and this to me is priceless. I go to bed trusting this discovery was meant to be now and not in a few days time. I go to bed determined to see John's joy at returning home once again.

Thursday 30 July 2009

Today will live with me always. Today John and I accepted, really accepted, he is going to die, and soon. It took John's wonderful oncologist of 11 years to say it before we believed it. Duncan has been at John's side since he was first diagnosed in 1998 and he has supported John in the way he best responds to: straightforward, logical, tooth and nail. He has given John every treatment and operation he can, he has fought for life always.

It was a conversation between two exceptional, strong and very good men. Two men who respect each other enormously, each never letting the other down no matter what was thrown their way. I had to battle my body's desire to openly sob and let the last couple of years flood out of me. It was a definitive moment in a long, painful and remarkable story of courage against the odds.

Today, reality sunk in, the mess made sense and I knew that what lay ahead was very different. We are no longer fighting for survival, we are accepting the inevitable. It's not something John and I do easily.

Duncan didn't want to give us a timescale as he worries that people focus on it, almost marking off the days on the calendar, but he knows how frank we are and that we want to know what to expect. No more than three months. Most likely to be caused by an infection or the increasing burden of the bone pain on John's body.

So here it is, the point at which we arrive: in black and white, no chance to blur the edges and disguise our escape plan. There's no ignoring it and it's up to the two of us to make the time we have together about living not about dying. I might be crying and sick to my gut as I write, but I will do this. I make my peace with this cancer. It is time to end the game, shake hands and walk our separate ways. You have had your time, you have made your noise and scars. You have won and we stop our fight against you. Now go and leave us to be gracious in our defeat. Now we will find the love and peace to silence you in shame.

John and I cried when Duncan left. John said he didn't want to leave me. I said he wouldn't miss me for long, not on a heavenly golf course surrounded with angels serving him Bud. I asked if he would come back as a friendly ghost and sit on my shoulder to huff at my ditsy mistakes and guide me the right way when life posed a challenge. John is the logical, practical, solid bit of me. He is the no-messing, say-it-as-it-is bit. He taught me to fight for myself and be strong, not to be so taken in by others. And he will always sit on my shoulder telling me so.

We had friends arrive as we were with Duncan, and I asked them to wait downstairs in the café. I then had the task of shaking myself into sufficient control to see them and ask that they hold off their visit for another day. I told them what Duncan had said but as always I tried to say it in an easy way. It's one of the worst bits: trying to make it comfortable for other people to hear the news. Truly I don't want to tell people just how much it hurts. I hope no one feels this pain.

Strangely John was moved from his private room to a ward of four. I say strangely for the timing from our personal point of view not from the view of hospital logistics – you never keep the same patch for long in the necessary juggling of beds and wards. We curtained off the bed when we first arrived and gradually settled into the new ward. The usual eyeballing of fellow patients occurred and I tried to be open-minded, with little success, about the noisy ned in the room. I wasn't in the mood for his loud-mouth slang chat and disrespect towards the nurses.

Once we settled in our clinical curtained box, we felt a surprising relief that we could now stop fighting. Throwing ourselves back at this monster was pointless. All we could do was be with each other, the kids and our friends. We talked again for hours about what we would do when John came home, the stuff that we used to take for granted. Those things you expect, so beautiful but simple they often pass you by unseen.

John imagined what I would do after he was gone. The ideas were varied. I'd be spontaneous and head off to some war-torn place to build houses or orphanages, I'd be happily eccentric in a house full of rescue animals, I'd find my artistic hands again and go to art college – a place I seemed destined for until my late teens. I'd need to learn to cook properly and I'd definitely get a scruffy looking dog and call him Hector after a dog I'd fallen for in an episode of *House*. John asked when the new series of *House* was out on DVD as he wanted to see it before he died. I cried inside at the thought I will never watch it or any movie with him again. I don't care what I'll do without John, I can't think about it. My life is about John and keeping him here. Without him it's nothing I can see.

I left just before 8pm so I could come home and talk properly to my mum on the phone. She's dealing with some problems of her own and is staying with my brother and sister-in-law for a while. We've been through a lot, mum and I, and it's hard not to have the room to help her through this time in her life. Everything is out of control and not just for me. The floor supporting my family is unsteady too. I feel numb.

Friday 31 July 2009

This morning I woke up feeling utterly horrible. The adrenalin is the gift keeping me going but is also the poison flooding my body. The sickness and shaking is getting worse while my racing mind is hard to bear. I remember about the melanoma, I worry that I feed it the stress it needs to grow stronger.

Outside it's a day for children being slathered in sun lotion before they play freely in parks and paddling pools, a day for BBQs and banter with friends, a day for cycling along the coast and stopping for a picnic, a day for pottering in the garden half-heartedly until the chilled glass of rosé lands in your hand, a day to see the colour of flowers, hear the songs of nature, a day to feel alive and well.

Inside it's hot and noisy, time is morbid. The minute broods slowly through us, each of its seconds an assault on our senses. The comforting aroma of hot coffee fights the ever-present linger of disinfectant and the occasional heavy odour of canteen meals being clattered along on trolleys to ungrateful recipients. The sun, free of cloud, blasts its rays through the huge windows, the magnified heat baking those trapped behind, reminding us of the carefree world it lights outside. The chatter of others, quiet and sad, loud and nervously obnoxious, the incessant bleep of the chemo machines, the ward phone ringing – the anxious relative on the other end desperately willing it to be answered – the metallic whirl of curtain rings hurried round the pole masking the groans of the patient beyond. Let us be home.

Tuesday 4 August 2009

I prayed last night that we would be allowed to step off the roller-coaster for our last months, weeks, hours together. These past days have been too much. The way time grew heavy and clingy in the Western, the relief at getting John back to the hospice to the welcome smiles of those beautiful people, elation that he may get home on Monday, upset that by Tuesday he was toxic again, the difficult chat with one of the doctors about how bad the cancer now is; it is in the final stages.

Among this I'm trying to arrange and rearrange a 50th birthday celebration for John. From one day to the next I'm unsure of where he will be, how he will feel or what he wants. First I arranged it at the house but as numbers reached over 50 I realised I couldn't cope with it all and look after John safely at the same time. Then I arranged for a room at the hospice when it seemed like John would not get home. Then when he looked better I arranged it for the local pub. In the end we have been advised to cancel the whole thing. It's too much; we are worrying about everyone else and not ourselves. So now if John is well enough then I will bring him home tomorrow and we will have only the kids and a few close friends round to see him. This is what he wants, this is what we can cope with.

My body continues to rebel against the stress. I guzzle pills for a kidney infection, racing heart, sickness and insomnia. From the minute I get up my heart leaps into relentless pounding, I'm sweating and lightheaded and genuinely scared I may just stop working at any moment. I burst into tears in the middle of the supermarket. I was buying party banners and plates for John's birthday, and when the checkout girl asked if it was for a special celebration I had no idea how to answer her. It just hit me that it would be the last time I would ever do this for John. Does this make it special or unthinkably sad? Will it make John happy or not? Will he find the huge banner his youngest daughter is making him happy or sad? Will he find the mad giant lobster-shaped birthday cake happy or sad? Will he find the huge piles of cards from everyone happy or sad? I don't understand any of it today. I just want him to be well enough to come home tomorrow so I can see his eyes relax as he settles in his favourite chair. John wants to be at home for his birthday on Thursday and for this reason alone I'm sure he will be.

Friday 7 August 2007

We did it. He was here. He was slightly out of it but he was here and happy.

It wasn't easy: getting home on the Wednesday afternoon, trying to get into a routine with John's care and meds, trying to welcome the guests in between me being sick in the loo. John did what he needed to. His daughters and friends have the memory of it. So it is worth every ferocious beat of my heart. His strength astounds me. He is the most inspiring, incorrigible, proud, solid brute of a man I have ever met.

Now the birthday is past we can find our peace. The meds are settling and John is regaining his clarity of thought. Claire is here in the morning to do the syringe driver and in the afternoon to check on us. We have emergency numbers for everyone we can possibly need to talk to. My spreadsheet and I are in control of all the scary meds, which I dish out four times a day plus all the breakthrough injections. Marie Curie places a nurse with us overnight to allow me to rest. So, it will all be ok, won't it?

Monday 10 August 2009

Thank you, thank you, thank you for this day. We have found a way to our island again. I am regaining my strength, John is returning to John.

The two of us, our trusty wheelchair – it looks like it needs an MOT but it can shift with my determination behind it – and our bag of emergency meds got in the car after lunch and med time and headed to the village's golf course. We parked the car and I unbundled the wheelchair and helped John and his pressure cushion into it. And off we set. It took us a while to really set off, John had a few golfers to watch first, but when we did we lost ourselves in the nurturing of another perfect summer's day.

As we trundled up the road, laughing about the slightly unnerving sound of the wheels struggling to cope with me shoving the chair, and John, up the long slow hill, our words flowed freely.

I asked John if there was anything he had not done that he wished he had. He said not much, that he'd lived such a full life, travelled a lot, been irresponsible, responsible, lived being naughty and self-ish, and lived being loving and protective. John's 50 years have been packed solid with experience and living, whichever way we look at it. There were two 'still-to-do's' however.

The first is very John, brave but miles away from the realms of normal expectations of the achievable. Doing a proper downhill ski jump I feel is something he will just have to miss doing. Trust me, if he thought there was the slightest possibility he could try it, even in his current physical state he would.

I managed to turn his focus to the second to-do. He has always wanted to play a round of golf on the Old Course at St Andrews. We have stayed in the Old Course Hotel a couple of times during which John was glued to windows or sitting outside watching players make their way round this historic and magi-cal place. My original plan for John's 50th was for us to spend a few days at the Isle of Eriska Hotel near Oban before heading to the Old Course Hotel for a couple of days. There he would play a round with his golf buddies and we would chill out in our beloved St Andrews. Then finish our trip with a stay at Loch Tay – the other place most likely to allow John contentment. We discussed whether any of this is still possible. We need a nurse to be able to change the syringe driver each day and we need to be close to hospital care. We need to have a shed load of dangerous drugs in our possession and we need to be blinking brave. John is sad but not desperate in admitting he has taken his last golf swing. He can't stand without crutches and his bones are too fragile to endure such movement. But we decided if there is a way then we should still go to the Old Course Hotel so he can feel the atmosphere of the place and be part of the golf. I don't know if this is possible, I hope it is. We both feel excited about it and I desperately want to make this happen for John. We will talk to Claire and see what can be done.

Tuesday 11 August 2009

We talked to Claire about our hope to go to St Andrews. That was after much hilarity at John telling her to lick a battery. She was checking the battery of the syringe driver and John persuaded her that the best way to know if it still had charge was to lick it. The first I knew of it was a small shriek from Claire and bursts of laughter from both of them. Yes, John is definitely here with us again. I told Claire about all the times he tricked the kids and me into tasting chillies and the likes, not to mention all the sneaky nerve pinching of elbows and knees when we were giving him cheek. It was the right time to talk about us going away for a couple of days. Claire is going to look into the nursing care side of things and we take it from there.

Friday 28 August 2009

It's not the time at home we talked about, we prayed for. Our walks together, our time in the garden, get sabotaged by other stuff, other people. Our return home is as tough a slog as life in the hospital or hospice.

I watch you dying, almost out of touch behind a barrier of routine and other people. 6.40am I'm up to get a handover from the overnight nurse. I give you breakthrough diamorphine, have shower, get dressed, make you breakfast in bed. Help you up and shower and get settled, change the bed, Claire arrives at 10.45/11am, doctor follows most days at 12/1pm. I do the necessary housework, then make you lunch. I try to answer some of the texts. We have visitors, I make coffees, chat when you tire, make hints for them to leave. I do meds at 1pm then 5pm, I make tea, answer more texts and phone calls, take the call from the out of hours nurses. We do some paperwork, not daily stuff, the important stuff about dying that you want taken care of. All the while the home phone squawks… the mobile chirps… all the questions, all the questions, all the questions. It's not support, it's assault.

At 8pm we go upstairs. I help you get changed for bed, give you more breakthrough, the 9pm meds and we lie next to each other resting and waiting for the overnight nurse arriving at 10pm, dreading being apart. I do a handover and go to the spare room. For a while I lie and listen to the sound of a stranger in our home, then I down two sleeping pills, sleep little, listen for noises from you and get up at 6.40am and do it all again. And all the while the deafening noise of everyone else.

I did not sit still for the first two weeks. I got angry at people not understanding we want to be alone, that we don't have the means to immediately answer every question they have, to constantly update them, to pander to all their fears and anxiety. They don't see they are tiring John out, that the most important thing is John and making sure we prioritise the medical care and rest he needs. We don't get more than an hour or so a day together away from the noise of others.

So in week three the doctor said enough was enough and to keep people away. To be honest we have no choice, I have made myself worryingly unwell trying to keep everyone happy. John wants to be at home, he needs me to be able to care for him. Our close friends get it but others don't, they are too consumed with their own emotional needs, feelings of guilt, to see they are suffocating us. I have stopped replying to some texts now, passed caring what they think, I just want us to have time to rest and be together. This behaviour is not normal: a usually private couple suddenly swamped by visits and texts and calls, often from those we have not been close to for the last few years. Our good friends give us space, but others are selfish beyond belief. Seven weeks ago I was told John had days to live. This is a difficult, desperate thing for me and the people closest to John to get our heads' round. We need the space and time with John. What matters now is John, the kids and the friends and family he wants close to him.

I feel like I'm failing in some way but our Macmillan and Marie Curie nurses reassure me we are not alone. They've known patients who had to put signs on their doors asking visitors to stay away and others who have screamed at everyone to get out of their house or hospice room. To be really honest, dealing with everyone else is the worst bit of this. We're at the stage of leaving our own home to get away from it. We talked about renting a cottage somewhere so we can focus properly on John's care.

I'm tired of holding it all together; there is no escape. I took John to meet his colleagues for a lunch in Edinburgh and then sat in a supermarket car park sobbing until it was time to collect him again. I wasn't well enough to drive that day or to pretend to his friends that I was ok. People only see the time they are with John, they don't see what we go through the rest of the time dealing with pain, other people, practicalities, the things that absolutely must be maintained with precision to keep John here. I hope our planned escape is all we dream of.

We are going to St Andrews on Tuesday. We want it so badly but I'm scared too. It's a huge responsibility. I only want to go if John finds what he is looking for while we are there. Do not take it away from us with pain and emergencies. Please, give us this one last thing. I know we are on borrowed time, I know if this happens it will be a miracle. Please just give us this.

Friday 4 September 2009
Miracles happen. We stole joy out of sorrow and found peace. The days themselves are invaluable but the memories of them live as love in my heart forever more. I realise how lucky we are to have been given this time.

I admit it was interesting preparing for it. A suitcase full of ketamine and morphine – and the rest – all double-checked, triple-checked, by Claire and me. I booked us a plush car and driver to take us to St Andrews, part of the treat for John but also so I was always free to do the breakthrough meds. We packed in our clothes, the rickety wheelchair and our suitcase of goodies and off we set. Impossible to relax until we got there safely but as soon as I saw John's face light up and the tears glisten on his sunken cheeks I knew we were doing the right thing.

Room 268, a spacious suite with its vast corner windows over-looking the 16th green/17th tee of the Old Course felt to John like a dream come true. He settled in a chair by the window and watched golfers for hours upon hours as he sipped our favourite Chablis and in true John style interspersed it with the odd sip of Budweiser. I sat cross-legged at his feet cheerfully waving to golfers despite being in my cosy PJs. The nurses from the local doctors' surgery met us that afternoon to check we were ok and arrange timings for redoing the syringe driver. They were won-derful, and knowing they were there for us immediately settled my nerves. To our surprise and delight they told us that Dr Smyth from their surgery and Paul McGlynn from the Links Trust had arranged a special tour of the Old Course for John the following day. We could not have asked for more.

We were both excited when we woke up on the Wednesday morning, that of my 35th birthday, a day I knew I would return to in my mind many times over. I had everything I could want in that moment: John was happy and pain-free, well-rested after a good sleep and nervously awaiting his tour of the course. After an indulgent room-service breakfast John gave me a gift bag and card. He was upset he had not been able to do more; I didn't expect or want anything other than our time together. It was a gift of charms for my bracelet, which he had bought for me previously, each holding special meaning to us. There was even one with a lobster on it. Claire had helped him wrap them and look out a card when I'd been out of the house. John has done a lot of thoughtful stuff for me over the years but this took my breath away. After breakfast and meds, I helped John get dressed. He looked as he always did: mirror-shiny shoes, sharply pressed shirt, clean-shaven and proud. I even cleaned up the wheelchair so it didn't let him down on his big day.

We got a warm welcome from Peter who was the course ranger driving John round the course on the nicest-looking buggy I've seen. John sat up front with him and I perched on the back, one hand holding the side rail the other hand gripping the bag of emergency meds. I was glad they could not see me as I cried the whole way round. This, like the conversation between Duncan and John, was a defining moment. I could hear Peter telling John about each hole and stories of famous players. I could hear John's interest and laughter. I returned greetings to the American and Japanese golfers who cheerfully waved to me probably wondering who on earth we were. I knew they would have no idea just how special the moment they witnessed was. I will always remember the welcome mix of light raindrops and sun on my face, the noise of the buggy wheels on the gravel pathway, John's profound happiness. The moment itself and the memory of it are gifts that could not be bought or replicated; it is a joy deep in my soul that can never be taken from me.

John was exhilarated after the tour. No amount of hardcore drugs could mask his delight. We went to the Jigger Inn for lunch and replayed the event in animated detail. John heartily devoured a fabulous burger and chips and sticky toffee pudding with ice cream – plus a boost of morphine – while I relaxed enough to enjoy the best fish and chips ever. I thought the day could not muster more happiness for us but it did.

John decided he wanted to get me a present that I could keep with me always, one that would remind me that miracles are possible and to live in each moment. A watch seemed fitting, and a watch it was. The elegant lady who served us in the jewellers, the lady who listened with impressive composure and warmth to our story, is called Elaine. She was wonderful with John, who was emotional and raw, and with me – I did not know what to do with myself. I will go back one day in the future and tell Elaine just how much she added to this treasured moment. In the evening we tucked into a room-service meal and champagne and drifted happily through hours of watching golfers tee off at the 16th. It is the happiest and saddest birthday I have had. It is the last birthday I will spend with John. And what a way to do it.

We had another restorative night's sleep and spent the Thursday eating, covering miles of pathway round the Old Course, and even took afternoon tea with champagne. More impressively we managed to get both of us in the huge Jacuzzi bath while keeping the syringe driver and John's bones safe.

The trip is packed with one marvellous memory after another but one in particular really rocks; it shouts 'John at his true best'. After we had lunch at the Jigger Inn on my birthday John told me there was something he would like to do. Something he must do. I was a little nervous but agreed to help him do whatever it was. Thankfully it was achievable, just, without injury.

I trundled John in the trusty wheelchair along the path that runs closest to the iconic Swilcan Bridge on the 18th fairway. I gave John a boost of diamorphine and handed him his crutches. He got up onto them expelling the aftershocks of each pain searing through him. Once he was steady and we thought there was enough of a gap in play to accommodate our tentative adventure we set off across the course towards the bridge. John's body was rebelling against each move he made but his will was more defiant. Whether we needed an ambulance to get him back off the bridge or not didn't matter; there was no stopping him. And there in the sun, in this historic place so special to us both, John did what many famous golfers have done before him. He took his official retirement from golf by standing proudly upon the Swilcan Bridge. It is there on that small, ancient, humble stone bridge that I finally capture the beauty and strength of this man. I know many great men have stood on the Swilcan Bridge but I doubt it took any such bravery and determination to do so. I love this man, I respect this man, I do not want to be without this man.

Monday 7 September 2009

I cling to thoughts of St Andrews. It was hard to leave its sanctuary. Our arrival home on Friday was chaotic. I was glad to see
Claire when she appeared moments after us, desperate to tell her
how well it had gone and feel her support our transition back to
reality. Lovely birthday presents from friends awaited me, and in
the afternoon Eleanor, our exuberant and utterly smashing Marie
Curie nurse, looked after John so I could cure my dark roots and
split ends at the hairdressers. It should all have been a real treat but
the stress of coming home to messages, mail, a ludicrous phone
bill, unpacking, sorting meds, groceries, while trying to make sure
John settled home took the edge off any time out. After a fraught
first day back we vowed to keep St Andrews alive. Over the weekend we hid from most of the noise, instead rekindling the peace we
found on sunny paths through majestic fairways. We trundled up
the roads surrounding the golf course and were quietly us.

We have our nights alone now too. I stopped the overnight
Marie Curie nurses before we went on our trip. A difficult decision, advised against by others. They are remarkable people doing
a delicate and crucial role, and their help is invaluable. They are
selfless in their giving. Our truth is that we want to be together,
alone. We want it to be us in the night, we want it to be me comforting John when the pain jolts him out of sleep. It means I can't
take the sleeping pills, that I must be alert. Somehow my body
is supporting this and my mind is sharper than ever. I want it so
much and I know what John needs more than anyone else. We lapse
in and out of sleep but if he moves or groans I waken and rest
my eyes in a steady gaze at his chest rising and falling. I have the
breakthrough meds ready and I know before it happens when a bad
episode will hit him. We are a single unit now, seamlessly in tune
with one another. Whether I'm giving John meds, helping him
stand or wash or eat we don't need words of explanation between
us. I never realised that such profound closeness is possible with
another person.

With the closeness comes the ability to deal with all the sensitive subjects, the ones you expect to reduce you to quivering wrecks, in a composed and coherent way. Perhaps it's because I understand John's no-messing 'here's what I want' attitude. I know already, however, that carrying out some of John's wishes after his death will not be without pressure. There will be noses out of joint. I need not worry about that: 'We are the two who have been in the thick of this for years and as long as we know what's to be done everyone else can sod off.' In theory this is how I should feel. I know I will not.

I'm clear on the formal will protecting the kids, on certain items going to certain friends, on where and how John wants his ashes scattered, the memory boxes we need to make up for the kids, the bench on the golf course and the songs to be played at his funeral. The actual funeral has been the tricky part. In John's words: 'I'm not that interested in it, I don't like funerals, don't want one. As long as I'm cremated and my ashes are where I want them to be then I don't care.' After I highlighted to John that other people who love him will care, we had the debate about whether it should be a religious or humanist service. In the end he felt comfortable with neither. On one hand he is not actively religious though he does believe in something and his guiding light has always been his step-grandmother, a kind and loving woman who was every inch the believer and whose bible John wants placed beside him in his coffin. We have arrived at a position where the hospice chaplain assures me they can do a service that encompasses elements of both a traditional church service and a humanist service.

Finally is my promise to John to do certain things for us and for me. Most of it is about me being true to myself, leaving the investment industry to write on subjects I genuinely care about, to stop worrying what everyone else thinks. John's main request is formidable in its magnitude, or it certainly is for a beat-up, exhausted and exceptionally private individual: 'You must tell our story. Promise me you will write the book. Really you are meant to, that's why you have the words to give to other people like us. If nothing else promise me you will do this.' I say yes to all, unsure that I will ever want to or be able to relive our story.

Tuesday 8 September 2009

I went to my check-up at the dermatology clinic today. I was scared. I don't have spare capacity to deal with my own problems. I have to be well. It felt strange to be on my own without John. I suppose I felt guilty at leaving him, despite the reason why. No point analysing my emotions just now, my logic is rotted by lack of sleep and adrenalin. I saw a specialist called Sheena who was about the best person I could have sat down in front of. She knows Duncan and the doctors at the hospice and sees what life is like just now. Her understanding and kindness broke through my defences and I dissolved into tears as soon as I left the hospital: relief that all seems ok — next check-up in three months — appreciation of the enormity of what I bear each day.

Sunday 13 September 2009

The rollercoaster is more unpredictable by the day. My brother arrived with my mum on Saturday as she is now looking to buy a house in the area. She's at a B&B in the village for a few days and then into a rental cottage until she can find a place she likes. The guilt is gnawing at me again: guilt that I should be looking after her, she should be staying here. Frustration that all this is happening at once, at knowing I can't give out any more than I already do. I think something will happen to me soon. The things I feel in my body and head are not sustainable. I bite my tongue a lot trying not to erupt at other people's demands and negativity. Some days the meds build up too much and John is spaced out and removed from the war around him. I need him here, to be at my side in all this. I need to feel our combined strength and knowing.

There is good stuff though, there always is if I look hard enough. A hug from my brother, some time out with him was comforting. John has had some random moments of extraordinary strength. The sun has shone brightly upon our expeditions in the wheelchair. On Monday John was out of his chair, up on his crutches to walk along the road through the heart of the golf course. Tuesday, the same thing but for longer, despite me begging him to be careful. I persuaded him eventually to settle back into the wheelchair until on our return journey we bumped into one of his friends. John was adamant he would walk alongside him. How can I deny him it, he looked so alive. His proud, smiling face is what I must root into my memory. The pleasure of sitting in our garden afterwards listening to the birds, talking about how wonderful it was that he felt well enough that we could go for dinner that night with friends. The reassurance of normality. I should not remember the trickster hiding behind it.

John fell twice before he would allow me to cancel our meal out with friends. The first time he was getting up from his chair and his legs gave way under him. The second time was more cruel. We had got him washed and dressed for our outing, we watched a hot air balloon going up from the field opposite, he looked happy with the freedom to choose movement and friends and going out. Down he crashed in the kitchen. It destroyed me inside. The reminder of the truth of his vulnerability destroyed him inside. His morphine-glazed eyes emptied and I knew it really was the end of our stolen holiday.

Sunday 20 September 2009

The heroic man who defied belief by getting up out his chair and walking only days ago has been barely conscious all weekend. The drugs are ramped up to worrying levels but it is that or the disgusting pain. There has been no sleep, just lots of distress. Frantic calls to out of hours doctors and the hospice to update them on John's condition, to get instructions about which tweaks I can make to the drugs and how to stop his anxiety. I need to change the bedding, it reeks of chemicals and sickness, it's the smell of cancer in our safe home but I can't move John, the slightest touch is too much for him. I tried to get him to swallow some of a nutrishake drink through a straw but his body would not allow it. I'm so exhausted. I'm scared I fall asleep and wake to find this body next to me empty of John. Please let us get through to tomorrow. Claire will arrive, she'll know what we should do.

Monday 21 September 2009

I'm angry with John today, angry with myself, angry at the situation. How can I feel anger towards a dying man? He doesn't remember the weekend, he told me so after demanding breakfast. He doesn't remember the terrorising pain, his barely conscious state, me having to force feed him his meds and beg God to keep him alive. No, all he knows is that he is not having this, he's not going back to the hospice yet. By lunchtime Claire and I had got him washed, dressed, downstairs and in his favourite chair at the computer.

Our doctors spoke to John weeks ago about where he would like to die, how he wants things to be. He does not want it to be in the house where we can't control things as well, where there is likely to be more pain, trauma. There has been too much happen here already, on this I agree. I want John to be as comfortable and peaceful as possible. He has endured so much, more than is imaginable, he deserves the end to be as calm as possible. The doctors are suggesting his return to the hospice. We know what this means, neither of us can comprehend the reality. It is time. I can hardly breathe.

We know that the last few weeks are a miracle, that no medical person around us can believe it, but it does not mean we are ready. So now John is fighting against it and I know this is the wrong thing to do. He will hurt himself and me, and everyone who loves him, more if he does not get the help we need. I know I have been blinkered in my determination to keep him here, to give him his time, but I know this weekend has tortured me. Now I too need help. I can't hold John's life in my hands any more.

Thursday 24 September 2009

We made the decision to move John back to the hospice. A decision that has broken all our hearts. The only way I have been able to accept supporting it and asking John to agree to it is to make the decision black and white: do we want John to be more comfortable? If we do he has to get the help of the hospice doctors. The side effect of another increase in the Ketamine is unbearable mental anguish for John. I have spent hours, days, trying to comfort him and stop his relentless tears. It is not possible to reason with him, the drugs are blinding him. I can't bear this any longer, to hear him beg me to let him die.

With Claire and Elliot at my side I told John we had no option but to get him to the hospice so they could rebalance the meds and let him regain his clarity. He told us all, when he could, that this was the most important thing for him: he accepted that he has lost his physical freedom but he did not want to lose his mental freedom until he absolutely had to, at which point he would not want to be alive. I know that only the hospice can administer and change the drugs in the way and with the frequency that John now needs to find this mental independence. But knowing this is the right thing to do does not make it any easier. I am accepting that John will die soon. I am now at my most alone, most scared.

Friday 25 September 2009

I can't rid myself of this emptiness, it consumes me. Already I feel it and he is still alive. The ambulance drivers secured him in a chair and took him out of the house. It is the last time John will see his home, be in his home. I stood on the front steps in disbelief that I was watching him leave. I burst into tears and asked Claire if he would ever forgive me for this. I know deep down it's not my fault but I don't accept that I can't prevent this all happening. We have always been able to stop it before. I can't comprehend being in this home without John. This is not real to me.

Monday 28 September 2009

John is settled back into the hospice. We both relaxed once we saw the familiar faces and heard their excited questions about our trip to St Andrews. Out came the photos, out came John's joyful recollections. They could not believe we had had so long at home; they expected a couple of days for John's 50th, if we were lucky. We had seven weeks plus a trip away. I understand how lucky we are, really I do.

I'm thankful the meds are balanced enough to deal with some of the pain while retaining John's awareness. He is making the most of his last conversations with his children, friends and sisters. There have been cross words from me to others, my plea to ask them not to tire him out so much. I understand their own desperation to grab as much time as they can with John but the more tired he becomes the faster that time will lessen.

We have had difficult, frank conversations with the doctors about when they will next need to increase the meds and what this means. It amazes me how together we can both be, even when discussing the realities of DNR and how John's organs may shut down due to the weight of the meds — though the doctors concede they are dumbfounded by how strong John's heart has remained despite the attacks on his body from the cause, symptoms and treatment of his disease. I read all I can about dying, ask the nurses the questions I need to. It helps a little to prepare my mind in this way but it's difficult to believe when he looks so alive.

I hear the voice of our wise friend Darshi, the knowledge he has shared with us in person and by email, all unobtrusively, peacefully. His pure and definite words have supported us far more than the louder, broken noise from others. He was a client of John's for years, then a friend, now the guide helping John to leave, free of anger, of fear; helping me to trust that I have the courage to love John enough to let him go, knowing he will not turn back. The enormity of this crossroads is overwhelming: when I am able to let John know that I am ok, and that I will continue to be ok without him, then he will feel he can leave. And I will face my aloneness. I know I love John enough to do this. I know it won't be long. I know I must accept it.

Thursday 1 October 2009
I'm trying to keep writing, I know I need to talk to someone for my own sake but my mind is numb to protect me. John was getting an intrathecal inserted at 9am. The meds are not keeping on top of the pain. The hope was that the intrathecal would channel the drugs directly into the spinal canal and closer to the nest of John's worst pain. The doctors who performed the procedure were personable and hopeful and thankfully free from the barriers of egos and jargon. I appreciated one of them taking the time to fully explain the intrathecal to me: it's not often a senior doctor hand-draws you a sketch of exactly what they are about to do. Their desire to help John was genuine and their frustration as each attempt failed was clear for all to see. It should have taken half an hour. It took three hours. Three bloody hours they worked up and down his spine trying to insert it, three hours we were all in that baking hot room trying to reassure John and settle him while his body endured more trauma. Three hours of stress with no real benefit at the end of it. The disease is too progressed, the bones and gaps between them are just not as they should be. It's not their fault, they could not have tried more than they did. It's just a sign of how advanced this shadowy creature has become.

Thursday 8 October 2009
It's hard to distinguish which day it is now. I feel at a distance to real life, as if I'm in a separate room watching it reel out like a movie. The routine is there again: getting John his favourite food, juice and coffee, helping him wash, answer texts, arrange

visitors. But he retreats more each day, his mind is gently walking away from us. I move away as he does, trying to find shelter from the storm I see on the horizon. We said our goodbyes in St Andrews. I must be thankful for this miracle and I must let him go. I must love enough not to cling to him now. It is against everything I feel in my body, heart and mind. I want to scream and claw and hang on to every last breath he takes.

I walked in to John's room this morning to find him not straining in bed but sitting up in his chair washed, dressed and the perkiest I have seen him in days. I burst into tears. I couldn't believe my eyes. The nurses realised it was a mistake to let me believe the false hope of the moment. They quietly explained it was an artificial high from another boost to the Ketamine. I'm glad that John's closest friends see him today, that he has the energy to chat to them as the man they know. To me it's a sickening reminder of what could be, of what should be. Dying disorientates those watching it as much as those it takes.

Saturday 10 October 2009

I'm in the room with John, writing on the notepad we use to play noughts and crosses and figure out visiting times. Since yesterday John has been drifting in and out of consciousness. I know it won't be long but the doctors say it could go on for days. He can't speak now but they tell me he can still hear.

I talk to him about when we first met and that funny moustache, our holidays in Loch Tay, our boat trip in Croatia, our favourite times at home, how proud he makes me and the kids, how much of his character they will carry forward, what kind of dog I should get, all the times I embarrassed him on golf courses, all the things I'll get wrong around the house when he is not here to keep me right, the doctors he has amazed, the people he has inspired, how he will enjoy the golf courses in heaven, the rollercoaster we have been on that's forced life through our lungs each and every day, how it was our solidarity in fighting to survive that seeded our untouchable love and how I will share it in everything I do. How I will miss my outstanding, stubborn, clever, self-righteous, inspirational, infuriating, caring, thoughtful, cheeky, loyal, invincible Lobster more than my mind, heart and soul can inhale.

Sunday 11 October 2009, noon
John took his last breath at 1.20am. He was peaceful. We were alone and I held him in my arms. I felt him go.

I desperately search to sense him beside me. The physical does not matter if I can feel him in each breath I take. There is nothing. There are no words for this bottomless void in my soul. Even if there were it is not right to share them. It can only be an unspoken knowing between people who have felt it.

John found his harmony. John's pain is over. John is free.

part two
doing what was expected

Sunday 11 October 2009 midnight

My mum took me back to the hospice this afternoon to collect the death certificate and John's belongings. In the callous deception of an automatic moment I felt my heart leap as I walked towards his door. I fully expected to swing it open and see him sitting upright in bed drinking coffee and being cheeky to one of the nurses. I could hear him call on me and feel his lips kiss my forehead. I was stopped in my tracks, and when I saw their faces, of those who cared so well for him and for me, I tumbled out of the dream into the repulsion of truth.

I'm thankful to be numb, I am hopeful the tight pain in my chest will transpire into something to take me out of this no man's land into peace with John. I feel no awareness of myself, no desire to be. I don't hear the birds sing, or feel the warmth of the sun. I am scared to close my eyes; even if I sleep I will wake to the force of reality thrashing through me.

Monday 12 October 2009

Today something – John, me, the need – has slapped me round the face and told me to pull myself together this week, things need to happen. The texts keep gnawing at my awareness, all the questions about when the funeral will be, what the arrangements are. How am I meant to contend with this now? Between mum, John's business partner Paul and information from the hospice I have a list of what to do. I hope to be through these next few days in a fast blur and then be alone.

Paul and I went to the funeral directors to discuss the arrangements. The funeral will be on Friday. I know I just need to get through this week and the funeral in the composed, presentable manner that John would want. The funeral is a necessity for others. Just get through it, shut my barriers down, smile on, get through it.

Composure did not grace me this morning, not that it mattered. I was on my own as I looked out clothes for John. It will need to be perfect, as pristine as it would be if he dressed himself. I knew the suit, the shirt, the tie, the cufflinks, the tie slide – such an old fashioned touch but one John insisted on – he would choose. The shirt was already ironed to an impossible stiffness but I did it again to make sure the sleeve creases could cut through butter. I polished the cufflinks and tie slide, picked fluff off his suit and polished his shoes so brightly it would make my granddad smile down upon me. That thing with the shiny shoes, something I love so much. The memory of Grandad letting me help him polish his shoes in the garage, the smell of the polish still now whisking me back to the safe adoration I felt for the other proud man in my life.

It was to my horror, and Paul's – and admittedly later to much laughter from us both – that the funeral director informed us there could be no shoes on the body for a cremation. Impossible, John would not be seen dead, quite literally, taking his final bow without his signature shiny shoes. Initially I thought I ought to change plans to ensure there were shoes on John's feet but then John's certainty about being cremated, not buried, drew me back to logic. There are lots of things to do this week and I feel unsure about most of them.

Once it's over then I can focus on John's proper goodbye. John's instructions were clear, so I can relax in the knowledge of what he wants. There are three main things I must do. First

I must complete the memory boxes for the kids and pass them over, plus whatever the girls want of John's. In the end John's handwriting was too shaky to write the messages in the cards he got for both the girls. After several attempts and too many frustrated tears we decided to get the messages printed inside the cards. It will be difficult but the girls are lucky to have this deliberate connection from their father, the words he wants them to read time and time again as they grow older. Being able to say goodbye is a gift.

Then the trip to Loch Tay. His dear golf buddies, Paul, Grant and Ian, are to go with me to Loch Tay to scatter John's ashes over the side of the magical wee stone bridge at Kenmore. Once we do this, I must give each of them the specific items John wants them to have. The boys are to play a round of golf at the nine-hole course which John loved dearly and then we will all get merrily pissed and tell stories, of which there are many, about John's escapades. I nurture and dread the thought of this trip. Loch Tay is our place. I have no idea how I will feel being there without John but I also know it is where I must say goodbye to him.

The third request is for a bench on the village's golf course. This will take some memory scanning from me as the night John finally decided where he prefers it to sit was a night we had both had more than a couple of sociable wines. I may need to chat to his friends and the course before I get this one right.

A fourth commemoration has come to the list, one that means a great deal to me. We met the affable, confident, sharp and quietly talented Mark early in our time here. Our big plans for changing the garden and adding decking and a patio needed the expertise of a trusty landscape gardener. So it was over a somewhat painful visit to my osteopath that I received a hearty recommendation that Mark was the man we needed. Major landscaping, one new decking area, one new patio and several years later Mark is still a regular visitor to our home quite often to rectify my disastrous attempts at 'green fingerdom'.

In recent times Mark has taken over the regular job of grass cutting, something John insisted on doing even with new hip replacements and fresh stitches. I secretly and nervously watched John from the windows as he limped round the not insignificant lawn trying to mask the confused look of pain and satisfaction. Over the years John and Mark grew to respect each other. They are different men, or so it appeared. Different paths taken but both built on similar values and similar levels of testing stubbornness. It was this that fuelled adamant debates around the logistics of building 'stuff', the length grass should be cut to – John preferring an army style scalping, Mark a more empathetic length to encourage sustainable health – as well as many a friendly man-to-man chinwag. Mark has seen John and me at our best and at our most vulnerable. Like district nurse Claire he is someone who, although inadvertently due to our initial need for his professional services, has become part of our home and someone we feel safe being ourselves with. Mark's request to plant a tree for John in our garden and his suggestion we could perhaps scatter some of John's ashes before doing so didn't cause me to think twice. Perhaps not a request made by John but one I know he'd puff up his chest with pride at.

For now I must try to close my eyes and escape the endless whirlpool of practicalities. They are a welcome distraction but an exhausting one.

Thursday 15 October 2009

I saw John today, in the coffin at the funeral directors. I've wondered before how this affects people, why they need to see the body of someone they love after they have died. To me it's not them, they have gone. My experience today only confirmed how I feel about this. I'm closer to John talking to him in the house, or at the top of a hill. John was such a force of life, the vacant body dressed in his clothes was far removed from his being. Is this the point, to be sure they have gone?

I put the things in the coffin that I wanted to and left shortly after. His youngest daughter amazed me; she sat and spoke to John for a long time. I see his strength in both his daughters and I know they will be as proud of their dad in ten, twenty years time as they were when he was strong and loud and swinging them round the garden by their ankles.

Paul and I also saw the Chaplain. I requested funny anecdotes from the kids and John's best friends and, together with something I wrote, gave them to the Chaplain. We spent a lot of time with him conveying what John meant to us all. I explained we wanted a good measure of humour and words specifically about John's character. Hymns were ok as was some religious sermon but not too much. It's difficult, the Chaplain John spent most time with at the hospice has since retired. I hope it's ok, I need it to be. At least the songs are sorted, John was most adamant about the songs — as per that post-it note I found what seems a long time ago. For his friends: 'IF' by Pink Floyd. For his sisters: 'You are my sister' by Anthony and the Johnsons. For his two girls and me: 'Run' by Snow Patrol. For us: 'Caruso' sung by Pavarotti.

Tomorrow it is. I know I will not sleep but I don't care, this feeling of raw fire inside me is part of who I am now. I hope the bloody clock comes tomorrow morning. I obsess about it but it's important. It's the large clock that hangs above our oven that stopped just after John died. I tried changing the battery and fiddling with the mechanism but nothing worked. John wasn't one for interior design, for picking furniture, or colours or paintings; as he put it 'I'm not sure when something looks right but I know straight away when something looks wrong.' This was a principle he applied to my requests for outfit approvals — yes my bum did look big in that. But John had positively liked this clock, in fact he chose it one Sunday when we were shopping. It was his choice, part of my memory of making a home together. When it stopped I felt sick. So in between funeral arrangements I have been trawling the internet until I found a replacement clock, the same as John's clock.

Friday 16 October 2009, John's funeral

It arrived, thank God it arrived. In black dress and bright red shiny high heels – I'll get to that – I clambered up my mini set of steps and hung John's clock. This was after I spent an hour sweeping leaves off the drive. I was looking out of the window at them at 7.00am and knew that John would not have leaves on the drive on such an important day. In jammies, boots and jacket I swept the drive and talked to John and felt grounded in the magic unfolding around me. The morning mist broke gently away from the fields and the sky turned from pink to bright blue. It is the day this great man deserves.

The shoes? Yes the shoes, and matching bag. In honour of the 'Lobster' thing. They are sassy bright red, patent stilettos. They are my shot of defiance and strength, the feisty bit of me John loved so much. Even better, a frazzled Gill and Nik have managed finally to get a hold of a red 'beanie' lobster to hide among the spectacular flowers for John's coffin. They are the type of dear friends where politeness and formalities are unnecessary. In seconds of meeting up with them our inappropriate story telling and roars of laughter fill the air. Gill and I met at college and lived together through-out many a student caper. That was before Nik persuaded her he was the right man to whisk her off round Australia before they returned to set up their own florist business. They are the most solid, suited, together couple I know, and John fell for their genuine warmth and cheeky camaraderie immediately. John's request for flowers from them was easy: 'Go wild with whatever you think suits, lots of those big bright red and green shiny ones I like.' The flowers in question are anthuriums, one of the many types of flowers that may not be considered conventional for a funeral. I certainly hope they will diffuse the solemnity of the whole coffin business with colour and boldness. It's John after all.

This is all the good stuff. Everything is organised, the clock is ticking, the drive is clear, the day is awesome in its brightness, my brother will be here soon. There is nothing I can do now but be there, rise above the petty family issues, which I fear may mar the day, and stand tall for John.

The problem is I can hardly stand. My body is in an uncontrollable mess. I've been sick so many times, I'm burning inside, my muscles are aching from the retching. My legs don't feel like they will support me. At least with so much adrenalin flooding me surely there is no way I can actually pass out. I took a beta-blocker, anti-sickness pill and an antihistamine, which sometimes helps take the edge off. There are temazepam and diazepam in the cupboard but I will not take them. I just need to feel those strong arms wrap round me, his lips reach down to gently brush my forehead and tell me: 'Toots, it will be ok, you'll do us proud.' I miss him.

God those words seem so insignificant, so inadequate. No one told me how this would feel, perhaps no one can explain this feeling. Of course if he were here he would drive me nuts, fussing over his shoes and suit and how clean the car was, checking his watch, telling me to get a move on. I wish he would drive me nuts again. I wish he would make me huff with frustration at his annoying particularness about every bloody thing. I would be so very proud to stand next to him. I must try to stand today as I would if he were here. If you are watching, Lobster, help me through today, someone needs to help me through this.

Monday 26 October 2009

I'm not sure where the strength comes from to perform my obligations for other people. I live in this private hell only broken by these false scenes of acting for the sake of others.

The funeral happened. Some parts went well, I suppose, other parts disappointed. It did not have the content we hoped, more religious than personal. Much of the words we asked to be included were not. The chaplain did not pronounce John's eldest daughter's name correctly, any of the times he repeated it. It was like a wedding – impossible to keep everyone happy no matter what. I got through it without losing my composure and was glad to be with true friends at the gathering afterwards. My brother and Kelly stayed with me that night and we drank and talked until the early hours of the next day. I'm glad it's over. If things weren't so complicated and if it wouldn't have caused ructions I would have kept the whole thing a lot smaller and more personal.

At least today I was able to hand John's daughters a copy of the stories we gave to the chaplain. I also gave them the boxes from John along with some old photos and certificates I looked out. It was an impossible day, what could I say to them. They've lost their rock and I know that they will miss him always. I want to sit them down and tell them it all, just how much happened, and how much we survived, how much we fought to keep him here. But too many things have been hidden to protect them, too many things gone unsaid. All I could do was hold it together while they were here and hope that they will be ok. I know they will be angry and hurt, I know they may feel some of it towards me but this is difficult to think about just now. I did my best for them, did more than that for their father. I have nothing left of myself to give right now. They took the belongings of John's they asked for, some of which were hard to let go of. I just hope these things remind them of the strength that lives inside and that they make him proud.

The phone has been ringing every night; mostly I ignore it. I know people mean well but I just can't talk about this any more. I'm exhausted pretending and I don't want to hurt people by telling them how bad this feels. The letters and cards give me strength. They began arriving a couple of days after John died. The most personal, poignant words given selflessly often from people I least expect. My body has given into endless tears day after day reading these lines. But knowing other people do understand this pain and have survived it gives me some hope I will get through this. Someone said to me that the best way is not to fight the feeling inside, or to try and fill the loss with something else, rather it's best to let it be and gradually it will tame enough to allow you to live alongside it, rather than fear it. The words that scared me were: 'It never goes away you just learn to cope with it.' It's impossible to imagine breathing in life alongside this feeling.

Thursday 5 November 2009

Mark and Claire came round today. Mark planted John's tree: a double flowering cherry blossom. We scattered his ashes, drank some of Mark and Shona's homemade sloe gin – a wonderful brew medicinal and lethal in equal measures that flows warmly from your throat to your toes – and I read some words.

Some of my own:

You drove me mad, you drove me to distraction, you drove me to the limits of my own survival. You are the best thing to happen to me. It has been an honour to love you and to care for you. You define who I am and I will love you always.

Some John kept in his wallet:

Night falls
But day dawns to replace it
Grief comes
But time will ease the pain
Life ends
But death cannot erase it
In memory
Love always will remain

Tomorrow is the trip to Loch Tay to scatter the remaining ashes. I feel sick. It has been a bad few days, my despair intensifies. There are people there, I sense their care and hear their words but I feel more alone. I feel removed from what happens around me, an observer to all this madness, anaesthetised in my bubble of loss.

I go through the motions of all the endless paperwork and financial crap. The frustrating phone calls to companies, to people who are lucky to feel the normal daily grind, at least they feel something. The discussions about my work, when I go back, if I go back, what next. The darkness, the emptiness in the house at night is the worst. I take the pills, drink too much and hope I don't wake into the blackness. Even in sleep the nightmares get worse. I'm awake, I hear the footsteps along the landing coming closer, I know they bring harm to me but I'm paralysed and can't help myself. John is trapped in a room and I can see him through the window he is on his side screaming in pain. I need to get help, break in, get him morphine but I'm powerless, helpless. There is no escape from this; both the day and night bring horrors and the real ones are as bad as the imagined ones. Loch Tay is our safe place but I'm scared it will intensify my loss.

Saturday 7 November 2009
Even under the onslaught of torrential rain, low, heaving clouds, and gusting wind there was light at Loch Tay. John was with me, all around me. I had gone to our safe place and there he was. Sadness accompanied us but much laughter too. It was how he wanted. The golf was played in the worst of conditions – though in a less stubborn or committed way than if John had been physically present – there was storytelling, good food and far too much drink.

The scattering of the ashes was a ridiculous affair. Trying to wave them gracefully over either side of the bridge was impossible. Some of John is in the River Tay, where he happily floats lord of all he surveys, but much of John settled in our hair and eyes and the velcro strips of our greatly needed outdoor jackets. We gave in to the humour of the moment and on that pretty but majestic old bridge said cheers to our best friend with our bottles of Budweiser. Somehow the laughter made me miss him more.

The next morning we met for breakfast. Feeling slightly awkward we tried to eat and chat our way through wearisome hangovers and our renewed longing for the fifth person not at the table with us – the one whose broad shoulders and confident voice would not have admitted to a sore head, swirling stomach or emotional vulnerability. Instead, we accepted ourselves as humble spectators as nature unveiled the type of morning that makes you thankful for sight and more thankful for memory. The heavy cloud was relenting its grip on nature's bewitching beauty, kissing the sea of lush forest as it lifted out of the majestic valley. Left behind was the utmost glory of Loch Tay, that bridge, our friend.

part three
stumbling into recovery

Once we had scattered John's ashes at Loch Tay I was alone. Even in the company of others I was locked up with my thoughts and feelings, in deafening aloneness. I hid at home, I hid away. I searched everywhere for John's presence. Time did not heal me or make me forget the loss. Time made me realise that loss could not be filled or softened. Once I stopped fighting the loss, I was able to settle alongside it. When I allowed it to be my constant companion it stopped trying so hard to make its presence felt. By letting it sit next to me, I could leave a comfortable space between us, enough to allow me to breathe my own air again.

Letter to John, Tuesday 24 November 2009

As I look at the golf course from this balcony it's easy to imagine you sitting next to me. Your eyes settling on the manicured fairways and greens occasionally distracted by the colourful parrots darting from one palm to another, your ears enjoying the glorious depth of the 'clock' sound that comes from a precise connection between driver and ball. You would love it. It saddens me we never made it over here with Kelly like we talked about. You two could have played golf while I swam and walked, then we would all go for fresh seafood and too much local wine by the marina. But we had our holidays, our perfect days, and I'm thankful for the touchable memory of them.

I wandered round the marina today and looked in estate agents' windows. I could run away to here, sell the house to buy a flat and the wee bar Kelly and I singled out as the ideal candidate for 'Lobby's bar'. The photo of you on the Swilcan Bridge would take pride of place, I'd have Lobster tat everywhere and do Budweiser happy hours. I feel I will do a lot of running away over the coming months but I know it's not the answer.

I'm not sure why I decided to stay on an extra few days after Kelly left. Part of it is that I can't face going home, I don't yet feel you next to me there. Part of it is that I have no idea what to do with myself. I felt immense relief when we first arrived: to not have your life in my hands, to be free of the meds rota whirling in my mind and the texts and phone calls nipping at my ears, to be far enough away to turn a blind eye to all the financial and practical stuff that is mounting up around me. It has been good to feel a bit of the old me again, to relax, to put the world to rights with Kelly, to laugh endlessly like school girls hysterical on tiredness and too many sweets. It would have helped me to live in these past few days for longer, but it only suspends the reality I must return to.

Even away from reality it is ugly. Too many tablets to get to sleep, to stop my heart racing, to keep my food down, and too much wine. I rest but I self-destruct too. I follow a few days of nurture with a night of drunken rebellion to shock myself to feel something, anything. But nothing. All I see is the chasm below me, all I feel is my uncontrollable plummet into it. I'm not scared though; I'm in nothingness. This feeling is worse at home where I'm closer to you, to us, in my heart but the physical distance between us is unbearable. I thought I would feel you beside me.

Letter to John, Thursday 10 December 2009

It was the only thing I felt certain of. Why is it not happening? Why can't I feel you with me? How dare you leave me at this time. After everything we have endured. I have given you everything I have, all my strength, and I need you now. Now you are free of your suffering help me with mine.

You are the only person who understands this, who knows our pain, our joy, our connection that was forever no matter what. Death should not break this. I thought it would feel stronger. I thought I would feel your strength wrapped around me. I knew it would hurt, of course I did, but I had no idea how much. I honestly believed I could not feel any worse than I did seeing you endure such pain. But it is much much worse. Unthinkable, indescribable, unbearable.

You knew that though; that's why you kept saying I needed to protect myself more for what lay ahead. You felt the unthinkable and you were scared for me. I thought I'd feel you with every breath I took and that with this I could endure it. My friend, my supporter, my protector, my purpose, how can I be without you? There is no reason, no will, no energy in me. For the first time ever I have absolutely no inclination to fight. And I have no idea who I am now. I'm just wandering lost in an endless darkness. My soul is numb, my heart hopeless, my body defeated, my mind locked down.

I am nothing, nowhere, just breathing against my will, going through the motions so others see what they want to and not what is there. I am my own fatality. I have died in some accidental way as part of a greater tangible loss. I am trapped in no man's land and the sign I need to find hope is not here. I want it to stop. I want to die.

Don't let me believe you would abandon me like this. I know it needed to end, the physical world that is. I know you hung on too long until you knew I would be ok, until you were certain I knew you would always be with me. Now that your physical torture is over, find it in your being to keep our energy alive. I need to feel it. I need our greater peace, or I will have lost to this lesser war inside of me.

Letter to John, Friday 25 December 2009

Merry Christmas Lobster. It's just you and me today. I'm snowed in, mum is snowed in and I declined the other kind invitations, not wanting to be the awkward widow forcing a smile in the corner. I just want it to be us today. So it is. You and me watching *It's a Wonderful Life* and listening to music in front of the fire.

You will not be happy with my dinner. The oil system is on the blink again so I can't use the cooker. I'm perfectly happy with my microwave sausage, mash and gravy and Christmas pud from M&S, and there's champagne of course. I know if you were here we would somehow be cooking full-blown Christmas dinner, all the trimmings and more just in case.

I admit to still feeling pissed from last night. I hope you saw us all next door, what a hoot. Your absence was obvious but we partied like you'd be proud of. I'm not sure you would have joined in with the karaoke but the banter was right up your street. Our bedroom was spinning when I opened my eyes this morning. I had a beroca and a beta-blocker and buckets of cranberry juice and then rummaged through a stash of the most thoughtful pressies. Then I made it through all the telephone calls, I think I did ok. I had a long soak in the bath and piled on cosy jammies – the ones that make you laugh out loud – huge socks, then an outer layer of boots, jacket and hat. I found a seat of two bin bags so I could make myself comfy by your tree to say cheers like we do on this morning. I feel you with me today. It lessens the anguish inside me and feeds my belief that I will once again see you clambering in the back door, jacket covered in snow, coal bucket in one hand, log basket in the other and the happiest, most satisfied grin on your face.

You never saw the snow so deep; it's captured our home in a surreal winter wonderland. I always viewed it as a gift from nature, a pretty white mask covering all the ugliness but today I see the weight it brings to everything it graces.

Letter to John, Sunday 10 January 2010

I'm sitting at the computer desk looking out at your tree. There is nothing that could inspire me more than seeing life that represents you. It is the straightest tree in the garden. Of course. The enthusiastic winds of the Borders have buffeted it ferociously from the first day it was planted but it always regains its natural presence, rooted firmly where it knows it belongs. It's pouring rain on your sturdy cherry blossom today, torrential rain. I know you'd still be out playing golf in this. I love you. I miss you in total: your good bits and your infuriating bits. I know, I'm surprised too.

Inspiration is in me but something more powerful is keeping it caged for now. I can't begin the words for the book; it's too much to put myself into those moments, happy and sad. I struggle to remember things with clarity. It's all fog and distortion. I spend hours wandering from room to room in our home seeking comfort but even the views and the birds don't gift me a smile.

Our home is driving me nuts. Is it you blowing all the light bulbs and breaking the dishwasher and washing machine to test if I remember what you taught me? Infuriating, even in your absence your voice is ringing in my ears to load the dishwasher a certain way, to change the timing on the drive lights, not to put the good knives in the dishwasher, to stock up on spare light bulbs. Why is it not telling me the important stuff like what the hell to do with myself, my life? I need a few nights with you sat at the kitchen table with a good bottle of wine to lubricate our thoughts and opinions on what I do next. This is the trouble, my confidante, my protector is not here when I need him most.

I resigned from my job, as I promised I would. I felt sad doing it, another loss. I care about these people; they have been good to me. The time off, the endless emergencies, watching me grapple to hang on to some sort of control, working too much and too hard in a blind fear of loss. It can't have been easy to observe; I feel our pain woke up fear in others. I know that world isn't right for me, but what is?

There are other offers, old friends, ones I trust, trying to help pull me back into the world, but nothing feels right. I know if I say yes to them then autopilot will take charge and I'll work myself further into the ground trying to fill the void with meaningless corporate pressures and obligations. But it's hard to walk away from my old life, familiarity is an easier route. I said yes to one contract but you will have felt Gill and Nik firmly talk me out of it. They are true friends, ones who know me – as Rose, not solely as your 'other half' or carer. So I respect their advice and get through one decision, one day, at a time. I feel our trusted friend Darshi by my side, his words helped you to leave in peace and now they guide me. He can see me, free of the past and the future, something I can't yet do. I still cling on to you as stubbornly as you clung to life. I think this trait, or is it fear, hurts us both.

Letter to John, Friday 12 February 2010

It is four months since you died. I'm yet to feel life flow through me. I was sick with knowing in the days before you went. I watched your every breath for hours, I saw you slowly leave your physical being. When you did I felt a searing desperation. I needed to pull you back despite the pain you were in. I knew it was happening but somehow it was still a shock. It wasn't possible that we lost. It was us against the world, remember? Indestructible, didn't matter what the doctors said. You were John Fergus, the one who surprised them all, should have died so many times and didn't, should have died six years earlier. It could never be over.

Now I'm in a place not of this world. One day raw, my soul bruised and bleeding, the next day numb, detached from everyone and everything with no care for myself. I am fearless, self-destructing, free from daily reality but trapped in the spin cycle of my loss. I lose you, my purpose, my routine, the self I became. I remain in this no man's land, drifting in and out of consciousness.

I went to the bereavement group at the hospice. It was tough, again made me consider the difference between losing someone suddenly or in a slow way. I am thankful we had time to find our peace, to say and do what we needed to, but I will always carry the weight of your long fight with the pain. If you had died suddenly you would have done so in the strong, fierce way that was you, but then you would not have had a chance to pass on your love and words to those around you.

At the meeting, there was so much misunderstanding, blame and anger from some, a lot directed at the hospice. I'm not going back for this reason. It is too hard not to speak out, to explain all the medications, symptoms, and the selfless care the hospice give. They saved us, not ended us. Those blinded by anger will realise in time and it's not right that I say anything. Our time was long, bringing knowledge and understanding. I can't imagine the shock if I lost you more suddenly.

Your clear eyes, your sharp mind, your dry humour, all died before you did, muffled out gradually by the drugs. But really they gave us those days, those weeks, those months where you were present. They honoured your wish to be alert, to be mentally independent for as long as possible. If we had a choice, I know you might have ended life differently, your time, your way. This would be fair. Everyone has a right to choose. The politicians are too scared of giving the choice and I understand why. If they'd seen someone thrashing to get out of their own body, begging to die or drugged into some numb acceptance, part of a sickening waiting game, then they may question their judgement. Then I wonder, had we the choice, would we have given in to the pain earlier and not hung on until the time that delivered you peace and defined who I will become. If we had the power would we have ended it before it was time?

I went with Paul to Loch Tay a few days after the meeting. He's the other partner you leave. He saw you, the best and the worst. He is lost too. I can be honest with him about my pain. It was too much. I was inconsolable. Months, years of wreckage poured out of me. I have been crying a lot since, mostly in the car or on the treadmill. They say it's good to let go but I don't feel better for it. Tonight was exhausting; I could not control the tears. I listened to 'Run', 'Green Eyes' and 'Caruso' over and over again trying to find an end to this consumption. I remembered the last time we danced in the kitchen, when you were well, when your strong arms surrounded me, when I thought you would live forever. I remembered St Andrews and our time at home, talking for hours, our walks at the golf course, leaning over and cuddling you in the wheelchair, kissing you on your head and breathing in every last minute of our time.

How did we come to find such strength with each other? We were not the perfect match. We were not 'the one' for each other. We were something else, something quite remarkable. Our pasts, our pressures, our insecurities, our determination nearly pushed us apart. The cancer made us walk towards each other again. In the end, we were more together than I thought it was possible for two people to be. Remember those words? Individually we are broken. Together we are fixed. Your logic and practicality, my feeling and creativity. Your disdain towards your emotions, my understanding of them. Our pain, our fight and in the end our harmony.

Letter to John, Friday 2 April 2010, Easter number four

It's Good Friday. Easter is without colour again. The snow returned. This winter has been the most cruel anyone here can recall. This latest assault has hit the farmers hard at the most vulnerable of times, so many lambs lost in just two days. The spring bulbs have been crushed at their pinnacle of bloom, the trees confused, the birds flapping madly back into survival mode at the feeders in every garden. I'm glad you are not here for this, not a happy face seen in days. We all need the life of spring, yet this year the extended winter mirrors the space I'm in. In some ways I'm numb to nature's cruel turn, I can't feel any worse than I do. Tuesday was different; there was a power cut late afternoon: no light, no cooker, no heat, my mobile signal was gone, my car snowed into the garage. I was shivering, too tired to build up the fire, sick with the latest bug taking advantage of my uncaring state. I could not feel you near me, this hurt most. I was asking you to be by my side but I felt nothing. It is one thing to be alone in the light and warmth but another to be so in darkness and cold. I don't want to return to that place, I must pull myself out of this emptiness.

I did some more running away, or rather following, in the hope of feeling something. It's a wrench to leave our home; I cling to it, to you, regardless of rationality. It's all I have of you and I'm terrified to lose it. I went to London for the weekend with Kelly to see her family, go to a show, eat nice food, drink too much wine. I could feel my body begging me to stop, flinching at the city's noise, lack of air. You know me, not a city girl even at my best. Two weeks later we went to New York for Kelly's birthday. You can imagine.

London seems like the west coast of Scotland compared to New York City. I was claustrophobic the minute I arrived. The madness of the place is fascinating but oppressive. How do these people connect to nature? Even Central Park crowded out my senses, motorways of joggers and cyclists. The magnificent trees, laughter-filled lakes, endless parkland framed by a monstrous grey skyline. Purpose built and I understand why, but it feels like a theme park not the flow of Mother Nature's hand.

The only photos Kelly managed to capture of me looking relaxed were by some of the park's trees and on the river walk in front of our hotel, the location of which was a blessing. We were on the tip of Manhattan looking onto the harbour, Lady Liberty herself, and Ellis Island. You would have been glued to the telescope – a lovely touch – for hours. Staying at the edge of the living movie-set, with the calm of the water ebbing away my tension, was what kept me sane. A patient Kelly had to take me on the river walk each day.

There were bits I enjoyed but I missed you terribly when I did. The loss overwhelmed me when we flew into Newark

Airport and I could almost feel you reaching over me in the plane to see the view and point out what each building was. The photo of me on the Staten Island Ferry seems wrong, you should have been next to me in that moment. You certainly should have been standing with us at the top of the Empire State Building as I ranted about the concrete jungle spilling out as far as the eye could see and wondered how on earth they support the required infrastructure. You would have gone on and on with all the trivia you retain about history, buildings, dates, specifications. We would have had to drag you from the viewing platform when boredom defeated our patience. The Irish Band on St Patrick's night in a characterful pub in the financial district would have had you belting your voice more freely with each new pint of beer.

The moments of shopping (there were many), champagne cocktails (there were many), and leisurely meals in trendy bistro restaurants (there were many), the odd cupcake and the Sex and the City Tour you would not have minded missing. Those were the self-indulgent girly moments, but I was not at ease the way I was in Portugal. I'm too physically exhausted, too emotionally raw to feel enjoyment, even in a place overflowing with opportunities to find it. I fear I did not give my best to NYC, even to its wonderful people, nor to my loyal friend who was doing everything she could to bring me back to life. I was an unappreciative traveller looking for something that can't be found anywhere.

So now I'm home again, relieved our place is safe but bruised from the thud of being slapped by reality. My sleep is a little better but pointless when it's filled with the nightmares. My heart is still racing priming my body to rush to your side, grab the hospital bag, get everything in place. I will never again be able to relax, my body is in fear, poised on alert, ready to fight. There is nothing to fight for.

The whole thing about six months being the point at which you feel better, what crap. Neither I nor anyone at the Maggie's Centre group feels a change at six months. If anything it's the point at which the protective numbness fades to be replaced by growing awareness that you will never again walk through the front door and hug me, sit beside me on a plane, be in your chair at the dinner table talking about our future. It's frustrating, this false target, as is the expectation of many others that I will step back into my old life. Perhaps I should sell the house and move back to Edinburgh, perhaps I should start running again, perhaps I should join some clubs, find more projects to focus on... well-meaning ignorance translating into loose, misdirected words which I hear as pressure, pressure, pressure. I absorb all this, multiply it by ten and feel I'm failing myself, you and everyone else.

As time goes on, sometimes it's the people closest to me who feel furthest away. The one person I need to speak to is not here. I'm so thankful for Darshi's ability to make me shut out the chattering world, for my friends who can feel what I'm going through, who are careful with their words, and for Maggie's Centre where I feel normal. These people are becoming the foundation of my recovery. I can't fail to be deeply saddened by other people's pain but I can relate to it and feel less alone. There are people in Maggie's group who are either side of me in terms of timescale and I can see that gradually people do move into a different space. Seeing someone who has been as raw and lost as I am now find themselves in small but definite ways gives me hope that I might be able to do the same.

Letter to John, Tuesday 22 June 2010

John Fergus
6 August 1959 — 11 October 2009
The strongest, proudest, bravest man we knew. A wonderful dad, a loyal friend, a loving partner. As passionate about golf as you were about life — in all conditions. You were our rock. You are our inspiration.

These are the words I wrote for your bench. A handsome, sturdy bench it is too, black wrought iron. It sits at the tenth tee facing that view you loved out past the course to the hills. Don't worry, you are looking first at the tee. I know you'd want to appreciate each set-up, each swing, each land of the ball, hear the banter of the four-balls and enjoy the odd expletive as balls see the rough. We got it placed the day before Father's Day. I'm glad, I think you would love it.

I've been busy since I last wrote, threw myself into a project – the work at the house, all the stuff we talked about doing but couldn't make room for. I hope you see how clean the drive looks now, I know it was driving you nuts and because of that it continued to annoy me. The log-burning stove was a messy job but the room feels right now, more cosy, more rustic, more me I guess. I added a couple of things from the local art gallery too, deliberately my taste rather than yours. The painters were here for weeks but they were a considerate bunch who did a thorough job and the weather was kind, so I found peace working outside most of the time. Then there was the conservatory roof – there's been a stream trickling down the back wall – and new carpet and furniture in the bedroom. Always my favourite room but it still seemed somehow 'medical' and sad to me, I needed to give it new life. I never stopped, trawling through the attic, cupboards and the garage, cleaning it all out. Paul helped me get to grips with a lot of the paperwork and with the garden, and of course Mark is making sure the grass is as you'd like it. Most of the repairs and improvements you'd love but I think my wild wallpaper in the kitchen is a rebellious statement. I guess that's a good sign – right? The house has a new lease of life, or at least its stresses have been eased. I hoped in doing this I would be cleansed, repaired, feel new but it matters not that some of the practical niggles are gone; nothing softens what is really wrong.

Physically though I think things are improving, tentatively but steadily. I have been getting acupuncture to help with the grief, the physical pain and my lack of sleep. Can you believe I can now get a few sound hours with no pills? It means I'm being sick less, feel more able and can think a little more clearly. I started running again and joined Helen's running club on a Monday night; it's often too much but I want to feel as if I'm getting stronger. Best of all are the twins – if only you could see the brightness in them and hear their cheeky laughs. You'd never think my brother and Lesley only took them on a few months ago. Their new family is good for the whole family; we needed a gift to come to us. Summer is ahead, if we get one; you know I'm always better in the lighter months. So maybe it can get better, maybe if I just keep functioning and doing positive stuff eventually I will feel something.

Letter to John, Sunday 25 July 2010

I hope you could see us all on Friday. What a glorious day for the guys to golf and see your bench. The course was bathed in sunlight and ringing with much laughter from the eager four-ball in your honour. Ian, Grant and Paul played, and Mike kept them company; I think he had his eyes opened to what a carry on you all had. I met them at your bench with cold beers and we all said cheers to you. We managed a few drinks before dinner at our favourite local restaurant, by which time the stories were free flowing for all to hear. We finished off the night with a few more unnecessary but enthusiastic nightcaps at the pub before we called it a night. The hangover was worth it; I know you were smiling wherever you are. There are so many stories to tell, ones that will stand the test of time. You remain vivid in many hearts.

I got an email from one of the American Football guys; he wanted to let me know that when he announced your death on the league forum there were five pages of condolences. I know you treasured all the letters you received when you retired as manager and I know in your heart you will have wondered if the passing years lessened peoples regard for you. You are still well thought of and remembered fondly. There have been so many cards and letters from your clients too; I read them to you and I hope you hear.

I'm still in the thick of dealing with all the practical and financial tangles. I'm so glad Mike and Paul are keeping a check on me, taking some of the stuff off my hands. I guess you had a word in their ears. They stand by you and for you, even now. I can't think straight and my memory is appalling, which makes it all the harder to deal with. In a way having to function to manage some of this stuff is a good thing, it means I have to get up, get out, get on. I'm thankful the insurance money for my skin cancer means I don't need to face moving straight away; the house is the only constant in my life. My situation would be far bleaker without it. How ironic: the cancer takes, the cancer gives.

I still don't know what to do about beginning a new career path. I'm sure if my body and head felt well my decision would be easier. The pain in my joints, neck and head seems to get worse not better, as if I'm covered in a layer of swelling. I guess my body knows what it's doing and at least now it gets some sleep. I stick with what helps: Darshi, Maggie's Centre, acupuncture, running, working at the house, walking in the hills. These feel safe and nourishing, free of questions, judgements and expectations.

Letter to John, Thursday 2 September 2010

A year ago we were in St Andrews living a day I will cherish always. What to make of this past year, so many extremes. It's a confusing day, I have the company of good friends, laughter, sunshine and thoughtful gifts but I'm raw and lonely. At 36 I live in the past or in an intangible transition as I move from who I thought I was to what is now hidden deep inside me. For now I relive those memories I'm lucky to have. I miss you John Fergus, my brute of a Lobster, more than I could ever have thought possible.

Kelly and I leave on Sunday, for Portugal again. I'm nervous about how I will feel physically and emotionally, homesick before I even go. But the point is to rest and recuperate. No pressure, just beach walks, swimming, dinners, reading books, spa treatments. Surely I can do this without my body's permission. Who knows, it keeps rebelling when I least expect it. Different niggles, bugs and ridiculous clumsiness, yes even more than my normal comedy with spatial awareness. I managed to give myself an impressive concussion a couple of weeks ago and was laid up feeling sick and exhausted for days. My brother, Lesley and the twins were here and I was gutted to miss out on the fun. I seem to be able to block any route to feeling enjoyment subconscious or not.

I'll think of you in Portugal, I always do. That happy week in Alvor, how proudly you would stride down the fairway we see from the balcony.

Letter to John, Monday 11 October 2010
As I lean to lift a match and strike it I see my hands shaking, I feel my heart pounding, my stomach sicken. I light a tealight and place it among many others on a circular metal stand. The flickering light looks beautiful against the muted tones of the old stone walls. I close my eyes to see you standing tall, shoulders broad, green eyes keen, polished shoes on firmly planted feet. I feel your defiance, your control, your unwavering protection of me. But I lose the gentle hug of the memory. I see you weak, writhing in pain, lost and exhausted, beating yourself worse at the will of your own retaliation.

I open my eyes to jolt out of the thoughts and huddle myself into a simple wooden chair at the back of the room. As I raise my eyes I look into those of a woman opposite and a man to my right. I can see the memories in their eyes too. I feel their loss and unspoken companionship.

I have come to this place today to feel safe, humble and peaceful, to a place uncluttered by life and other people's opinions. A place where I have the permission to be alone with my thoughts a

year since you took your last breath. I'm sitting in the Abbey on
Iona. You'd feel at home here. I feel its solidity, its history and
perseverance through the greatest of battles. The contradictions
of peace and war, love and brutality that etch it with character
and pride – that make it unforgettable.

The voice of Dark Angels was what finally woke me
Ten days after I wrote that letter to John I was sitting in Toftcombs House just outside Biggar, a town south of Edinburgh. I
was trembling with nerves and kicking myself for being so bloody
stupid to have committed to this course. Yes I'd always wanted to
go on it but that was when I was confident and well and focused.
I was now a directionless, nervous idiot sitting among a group of
very together, professional, confident people. Most of the students were from London, I was from a nearby village; most were
in the steady throes of exciting careerdom, I was bumbling along
hoping to begin a new freelance writing career, sort of, maybe,
perhaps. I was out of my depth. Really.

As it turned out, the writing course, Dark Angels, was the
firm but fun big-booted kick up the backside I needed to start
writing again. This particular course had found me, or rather
Stuart Delves, one of the tutors, had. I met Stuart a few times
over the years when our business beings crossed paths, though
our original meeting followed my colourful plea to work for his
agency. My admiration of Stuart's work has stood firm over the
years and when he suggested the course might be what I needed
to find my writing fingers I just said yes and hoped for the best.
I also prayed I would be able to string a sentence together by the
time the course date arrived.

I could hardly speak the day I arrived at Toftcombs. But somehow, the people, the way they teach, the unexpected exercises
they use, coaxed my mind out of survival and into creativity. The
glory of frontal-lobe living as I now call it. I was amazed how easily I threw myself into the quick-fire exercises and how happily I

poured out creative words I thought were far out of reach to my burdened mind. The course is designed to teach you how to use words more imaginatively in business – to engage with your client on a human, sensory level. It meant we all got to know each other fairly well. The nerves of first impressions were long forgotten by the end of Day One. Stuart and his fellow tutor Jamie Jauncey were open in their teaching and constructive in their feedback while the seven other students – each with a different story, a unique voice – were inspiring. I stopped feeling lost and finally found my own voice again.

I did write some pieces inspired by John but it wasn't until the last evening that I read out some words I intended as the opening to this book, the ones that you read in the first pages. The reaction of my audience, of people I had grown to respect and admire, made more of a difference to me than they will ever know. By reading out loud words of our story, words I had never shared with anyone, I opened the first pages of our book.

When I returned home from the course I finally confronted the one thing I knew I had to do but had been too muddled, too scared to do. I sat down at the pink laptop John bought me before he died, the gift that carried the dreaded weight of a promise, and wrote furiously. I could not stop. Not until my body began shutting down.

The final hurdle
I can't remember at which point exactly I realised that although my head and heart were regaining some strength, my body was shouting a loud, firm 'No!' at me. The running became a problem: one day I could happily churn up the hills for five miles; a couple of days later climbing the stairs was too much. There was the weird pain and swelling on my neck and head which Sheena, my trusty expert on all things muscle and bone, suggested was more than just muscle strain, seemed more like a glandular problem. Some visits she would carry out lymph drainage, which would

provide relief for a few days until I felt floored again. I remember her mentioning ME, as she had done before, and a recovery course in Wales that received encouraging reports. I ignored it all. It was in my head, I battled on.

At some stage I realised I should be better. The joint pain – to the extent I was sent for an X-ray – ridiculous sensitivity to hot and cold temperatures, loud music or sound, my hopeless stomach, my increasingly foggy mind, and the persistent flu-like symptoms finally persuaded me to at least go back to my doctor, Elliot. I explained that all these symptoms did not seem like a common part of the grieving process. I went for all the tests, filled in the lengthy diary questionnaire and heard from Elliot that it did seem that ME, or chronic fatigue syndrome (CFS) as they call it now, seemed like the culprit. I was referred for an appointment with a specialist at the Western in Edinburgh, which I was told could take months to come through.

Letter to John, Monday 17 January 2011

I guess you are infuriated at my lack of activity, you think this is just in my head. I keep telling myself it is, to get a grip of myself and move on, but the more I do the worse it gets. What is happening to me and why now? I hope you saw that I was getting better and how settled I was on the writing course. I hope you of all people see how hard I am trying. Surely I have done, and am still doing, my 'grieving time'. I feel that everyone around me must be thinking I'm just depressed and hiding indoors, retreating from everything. I dare not commit to seeing anyone or doing anything as I just have to cancel. I can't get anything done at the house, or write for more than a few minutes. The lack of mental clarity, the forgetful muddled head, the inability to find the most simple words, the exhaustion when I have to converse with someone is worse than the physical restrictions. Articulating answers to simple questions feels overwhelming and I long to seek refuge in writing but nothing comes.

I'm not sure when the first day was that I had no choice but to give in and go to bed. I think it was a couple of weeks ago after I got back from Chatel. My body feels broken, totally. My legs burn and shake climbing the stairs, my arms give in trying to open a jar. Standing, sitting, concentrating are all too much. Each seems like a mountain to climb, the very prospect of which brings me to tears. I have finally shut down. At my worst the days pass in a haze. I wake up and sit upright in the bed for an hour or so before I feel able to go downstairs and get breakfast, which I bring back to bed with me. After that I need another couple of hours' rest before I tackle showering. Then I head back to bed feeling like I have done a hard workout in the gym. Reading is too much for my head to contemplate so occasionally I stare at various telly programmes not really taking any of it in. I try to get some tea before I settle down to sleep for hours and hours on end. Some days I feel a bit better when I get up, but quickly my body starts shaking and I feel overwhelmed with weakness and know I have no choice but to stay in bed again. My mind is frustrated with me, ferociously stirring the thoughts, growing the feelings of guilt and failure. I don't understand this so I can't expect anyone else to. I just want some answers, a way to get out of this. Your frustration must have been so much greater than mine, I can't bear to think of it.

The physical recovery

It was not the start to 2011 I hoped for. The plan, how I love a plan and a list, was to finish a first draft of this book by the end of January. Instead words were out of my reach. January was a lost month, much of which I don't remember. I was desperate to find a way out of the mess, to be able to achieve something each day, but my body would not allow the smallest of tasks. I looked at John's tree a lot, feeling him frown back at me. I knew if he were here he would not accept this illness with its blurred edges and difficult diagnosis. Deep down I knew I invited it into myself, my body had been warning me of the problem for months and I had ignored it in favour of my adrenalin-junkie mind. I even went for ski lessons in December, despite my muscles begging for mercy. My desire to please, to not seem weak, was too compelling. It was madness, I see this now.

My mum and I were due to join my brother and his family in the Alps for Christmas, something we were all excited about. For many years my sister-in-law's parents owned a beautiful chalet in the village of Chatel, which they ran as a business up until recent times. Now they were looking to move back to the UK so had put the chalet, which was much loved by all their family, up for sale. We were all keen to have a memorable family Christmas and let my two nieces enjoy the magic of the chalet before it was sold.

My brother and sister-in-law are keen skiers and I desperately wanted to join in the fun on the slopes. I hadn't skied for 20 years so decided to get some lessons at an indoor ski centre near Glasgow so I'd be raring to go by the time I hit Alpine snow. The first lesson was a three-hour intensive beginner and while I was truly exhausted afterwards, mentally I was exhilarated by how well I got on and by the prospect that perhaps skiing could be my new hobby, something just for me. It combined the things I love: inspiring scenery, fresh air and exercise followed by good rustic food, excellent wine, open fires and a well-deserved sound night's sleep. I set my heart on taking to the skiing easily and having a fulfilling and rejuvenating holiday. Before we were due to leave I managed another one-hour lesson at the indoor centre and a couple of practice sessions. I was ill, really very ill. It was causing me to feel stressed and fidgety, which did not set me up well to deal with the couple of days before we left for Chatel, which in themselves were not entirely relaxing.

The worst winter in memory was blighting most of the country. Dealing with the most basic of tasks was a tiring challenge not to mention the added threat of frozen gutters, pipes, power cuts and the likes. Given the harshness of the previous winter I had prepared more thoroughly for winter 2010/11 by getting gutters cleaned properly, putting in a log-burning stove and getting my oil-fired heating system fully serviced in the autumn. But the day before our departure flight, the heating stopped working. We thought that once again water had got into the tank and had frozen somewhere in the line stopping the oil flowing into the cooker. But no, after several hours we discovered that a part in the fan was broken, a part that the manufacturer could not get to me for weeks. I was gutted. I wanted to go away knowing our home, John's home, was safe and warm and that I'd not return to burst pipes, freezing rooms and dead plants. I needed to know our home was safe.

£450 spent on electric heaters and a kindly pep talk from mum later, I agreed to leave the house in Paul's hands and still go on holiday and aim to relax. The stress was getting to me more than ever because physically I didn't feel I could cope with normal stuff let alone added hassles. In my mind everything was out of proportion and overwhelming and I couldn't understand why. The next morning I was a mess, being sick and shaking. I needed to sleep, not talk or deal with anything let alone travel, but the idea of not going was unacceptable, I had to. How could I not go and enjoy a warm family Christmas after the sadness of the previous year. I got there wearing the bravest face I could find and loved the place. It was all comforting natural wood, log-burning stove, pretty lights and amazing views.

I relished the first two days' skiing. My brother had encouraged me to buy the ski pass for the wider Portes du Soleil area rather than just Chatel, meaning they could take me on some spectacular runs. I found my ski legs fairly quickly. The first day I fell five times but I was on a red run. The same run the following day I had no falls. We were mainly skiing when my nieces were in ski lessons so I was only doing two to three hours, which was a relief. My legs were aching and I felt sick and shaky by the end of each run, but the enjoyment of being out on the slopes was addictive and I wanted to keep going. By the end of day two, after some one-to-one lessons from my brother, I was managing parallel turns. I was delighted with the freedom of it all. By the end of day three I had badly hurt my left leg and was gutted.

My brother and I had gone skiing on our own and it was a white out. I knew I'd struggle as I couldn't see the undulations of the slope and my confidence quickly diminished. My brother was very patient as I fell every few metres down the top part of the slope. Ironically the fall that hurt my leg was probably the least spectacular. It was a quietly nasty one, bad angle, tired legs not able to unrumple themselves fast enough. I felt ripping and popping, then sick fire up my gullet into my mouth. I knew something happened that would not just wear off, but pride got me focused on my brother who was waiting further down the slope. I clambered upright and painfully snowploughed down to him. I must have looked a little drained as he took me for a hot chocolate and offered that I ski down the short route back. I insisted we finish the longer run. Each turn was exhausting but I got down by whipping myself mentally; what a bloody idiot for falling, just carry on and it will be fine. Of course it wasn't fine and later that same day I fully cemented the initial damage when I lost my footing trying to pick up one of my nieces. That was the end of the skiing for me and the beginning of agonising limping everywhere supported by knee supports and lots of ibuprofen. I was deeply upset by the whole thing. To me it didn't seem too much to ask to be well enough to ski for a week without any issues – to feel well and alive and distracted from the past.

As it turned out I'd torn the muscles that run up the left side of my leg, beginning at the toes and ending at the side of the knee, where I damaged the adjoining tendon. It took four weeks before I could walk confidently on it, although even now it maintains a retaliating bite when I least expect, a valuable reminder of my stupidity. By the time I got home I knew my body was desperately tired and that it was no wonder I injured myself so easily. My muscles did not want to be twisted and turned repeatedly down a slope no matter how much my mind sought the distraction. It was only days after our return that my health deteriorated to the point where getting up to have a shower was all I could manage in a day.

I was desperately trying to do the right things to fuel my recovery. I was eating only vegetables, berries, lean protein and wholegrains, I stopped drinking alcohol and I was taking a raft of vitamin and mineral supplements. I finally listened to my body: when I felt I couldn't carry on, I stopped. I cancelled almost all my arrangements for work and to see friends. I accepted the abuse I'd done to my body and permitted it total rest. But I could not carry on for months like this, unable to get out to walk, unable to write. I'd spend an hour each day, more than I could comfortably manage, researching the internet to find out more about conditions like ME/CFS, symptoms and recovery. I dealt with John's cancer with information and I'd deal with my own illness in the same way. With better understanding came an openness to try anything and everything that might help me feel well. My appointment with the CFS consultant at the hospital was not until the beginning of April and I was keen, determined, to try as much as possible in the meantime.

After seeing a nutritionist I changed my diet to only homemade, wholesome warm meals, no dairy or wheat, two healthy snacks a day. With Darshi's help I learnt how to quiet my mind, to be present and meditate each day. I went back to acupuncture, booked in for massages and got herbal teas and oils to help calm my system. I began learning the Alexander Technique to ease the aches and pains on movement and resting. All these approaches and treatments made small, tentative improvements but fell short of tackling the root cause of my disease. When I applied for the course Sheena had mentioned in Wales – the Energy Excellence Course run by Amir Norris – I felt everything was riding on it. These three days in Swansea had to show me how to heal my body.

Letter to John, Monday 14 February 2011

I think about you, about us, about the depth of togetherness we found, the fragility of the time we shared. Sometimes I still think of your pain. It will happen in the most unexpected of places. A stranger in a wheelchair can do it. One time I was in a restaurant at a garden centre with mum. I went to collect our meals and as I returned I passed a man at a table close to us, he was in a wheel-chair and he had those eyes. You know, those eyes that used to mask your true ones? Eyes with pupils constricted by drugs, a empty, numb look, their owner sitting on his own waiting for whoever he was with to go and collect his lunch because he was stuck in that chair. No one paid any attention to him. I felt him completely, I imagined the pain, the life that had gone before it, I saw the man that had been and the man that was. It's too easy for people to look past him. I only made eye contact for seconds but it ceased my breath, drew me back through the bars of the cell to helplessness. I was flooded with every bit of the physical angst I felt when I used to see your eyes look like those of someone else, taken by the morphine to a distant place. Two women bustled to his table with food and drinks and settled next to him. I hope they never hurt as I do.

It is getting a bit better. The flashbacks attack with less fre-quency and force. When they come I observe them and then dis-miss them. My thoughts have tormented me for far too long, pre-venting me from seeing where I am right here, right now. Pain, regrets, guilt, unloved achievements, an over-imagined future. It is good to rid myself of the weight of it all.

I choose to fill my mind with healthy food. Not the pain of the cancer but the love and strength it gave us. The countryside that balances me, the new knowledge and perspectives that stimulate and nurture me. The physical, strong, well John, the one who is full of life, cheeky and caring, boisterous and infuriating. It's this John who I feel by my side, the other one is becoming more dis-tant. Like the Rose who was your carer, who lost herself in you, for you; she is drifting away. It is me at your side again. Finally I return home.

To fight, flee then trust

I was cynical ahead of the course, even after reading all the remarkable recovery testimonials of previous students. It was a long way to travel when I felt floored and it cost money I wasn't making. Worse – if it didn't work it carried the potential to make me feel and look like a total fool in front of family and friends. I already felt like an excuse maker and I didn't want or need to add to my paranoia or give others reason to question my health and judgement. My concerns were eased slightly by the application process. It was thorough, there was no guarantee Amir would accept me unless he believed the course was relevant to my problems and could help me. He tested me on one of the course techniques and suggested a range of helpful reading prior to arriving. I needn't have worried.

Alongside my treasured hours with Dark Angels, it was the most personally positive, valuable three days I had spent since John had died. Finally I made sense of what was wrong with me and gained the tools to help fix it. The trip away on my own also did me the world of good: a bit of space with only my own actions and needs to think about. It's fair to say that Swansea is not graced by an abundance of natural or architectural beauty but its wonderfully warm people and surprising gem of a beach made me happy, very happy in fact. The sun shining as if it was midsummer did of course help, as did gentle pottering round the Marina and long walks to pretty Mumbles. More, it was the definite feeling that I understood myself and what I needed to do to be well and at peace – physically and mentally – that marked it as turning point number two. In hindsight, if I could have gone to Wales before meeting the Dark Angels then I would have scribbled out these lines months ago.

By the end of the first morning I had met an inspirational group of people – the common understanding and acceptance was empowering – and avidly soaked up all the information about the function of different parts of the brain, how we establish neurological pathways and create chemicals in our body. The background alone was fascinating and I felt that everyone should know how to keep their reptilian brain in check and drive from their frontal lobes more often.

I finally accepted that the gift of adrenalin, which had looked after me, and John, during a long, long time, was now my poison. Over the short term it was effective, the lifesaver it's designed to be, but I had lived poised in 'fight or flight' for so long it was the only gear my brain could find. I was still producing enough adrenalin to take on an army but had no need for it and so wasn't using it. The excess adrenalin is stored as lactic acid – a toxin to us – in the muscles and organs causing disruption to the body. The cycle is worsened as adrenalin is an immune suppressant and reduces our ability to process toxins. It's like a double-pronged attack on our core healthy functioning, with the result being weakened cells, a laboured immune system, sleepless nights, sensitivity to a number of external stressors and true exhaustion.

All my symptoms were explained, from high blood pressure to stomach problems, and from mental fog to sensitivity to noise and light. My circumstances, my need to survive, had conditioned my brain to protect and fight. Finally, sense, clarity, acceptance, understanding. A leap forward.

The rest of the time in Swansea we learnt a toolkit of physical, behavioural and neurological techniques to break the harmful cycle we were trapped in. We learnt how to control the adrenalin and to reintroduce our bodies and minds to a state of calm and growth. We were told to use the tools as often as needed for around four to six weeks after the course, at which point we should have done the necessary work to reach a state of natural functioning. By the end of day two I had less pain and more energy despite my body going into a mad but expected state of detoxification as the lactic acid left my system. It was hard work to keep using the techniques, especially if I was weary, but by the end of week two I noticed many more improvements: digestion working as it should, energy levels increasing, joint pain gone, sickening pain in my neck and head significantly reduced, muscle aches easing, sleep more sound, clarity of thought and ability to recall sharpening by the day. Even better when I felt a rush of adrenalin being fired I was able to nip it in the bud before it flushed through me. I was still nervous about committing to seeing friends socially but gradually I was stepping back into life. My days became fuller, more productive, more fun. I began to see things more clearly and feel positive emotion I thought was lost to me.

On the first Friday after the course I crashed and almost burned. Wiped out on the sofa. I was gutted, until I looked at what I'd done in the previous seven days realising that even a supposed healthy person might need a nap at this stage. I got carried away with my newfound energy as many people do after the course. It was a valuable lesson. It has taken me years to do this to my body and it deserves the time to recover fully, confident it is headed to better times.

In the days after Swansea I also attended two important hospital appointments. The first was with the CFS consultant at the Western. I was worried about being fobbed off with a recommendation of graduated activity and not much else. I was wrong. He was an impressively shrewd man whose warm nature and obvious knowledge made me forgive the lengthy list of necessary quick-fire, sometimes difficult, questions. He helped me further appreciate how and why I found myself unwell, was supportive and confident about my recovery and encouraged me to continue with the book. By this point I knew that on the days I wrote I felt much worse that evening and the next day. Emotionally though, I was dealing with the grief and trauma head on, I was processing it and hopefully putting it to rest for good. All the necessary bloods and samples were taken, physical examinations conducted and a follow-up appointment set for May. The consultant discovered a couple of mildly leaking heart valves, a surprise to me but not a worry, and high blood pressure, not a surprise itself though the levels did cause us to to raise eyebrows. Overall, considering, I was holding up ok.

The second hospital appointment was at the dermatology clinic. I was nervous for obvious reasons but again expected to be fobbed off, this time with comments about it being my responsibility to check my skin. Again my fears, as Amir pointed out False Expectations Appearing Real, were wasted. I left following a lengthy conversation, thorough examination and confident thumbs up from another shrewd but warm consultant.

I walked through the sanctuary of Edinburgh's Meadows back to my car with tears streaming down my face. Was I well, not exactly, but everything was falling into place to allow it. The final thing I needed to do was write the book, and now I felt I could. I knew that once I fulfilled this promise to John, to myself, I would finally be well.

So here I find myself, just weeks after the course in Wales. Each day I use the techniques. Some days I feel buoyant, others I struggle. Each day I walk outside. Each day I write. One day at a time, in each present moment, and I am almost there. It's eighteen months since John died. I still miss him. I think of him, to him, with him. Some days a reminder of the pain will take my breath away, others a reminder of our joy will renew me. I realise I needed time after what we went through to repair my body and mind; I needed professional understanding and help to stop them being prepared to fight all the time. More than anything I craved the room to quiet the noise of the past and of everyone else so that I could hear myself again. Now I have settled in this space the apprehension is lifting, the mind is clearing and what I feel is my balance, my natural pulse. I no longer miss John with overwhelming desperation, now I feel him at my side, our bond a consciousness inside me, a knowing of what endures in life. He is safe and so am I.

Finally… a good Easter

As I write these final words it's April 2011. It's the scene of a vibrant spring. Nature and its creatures are exuberant with life. I have never seen so many healthy lambs. To lighten the season yet further my dear friends Gill and Nik have just had a gorgeous baby boy. I remember the loss this time last year and wonder at the growth now around me. Life flows through and on.

I have just spent a lovely, calm, adrenalin-free Easter with my family. Who would have believed it? I potter in the garden a lot. It feels real. John's tree looks beautiful. I never thought of him as the double-flowering sort but the white petals of expression soften his rough bark, his forced uprightness. I didn't notice last year, but there's also a cherry blossom above his bench at the golf course. How much more you see when you are open to doing so.

In preparation for the course in Wales I had to write a list of twenty things I look forward to doing when I feel well. It was to be a mix of small daily changes and more challenging aspirations. Following is my list, and it is where I end this book. It is time for me to let go of this story and begin a new one.

The 20 things I look forward to doing when I am well

1   *Trust.*

2   *Free myself to live in the moment.*

3   *Believe in the book: complete it with ease and publish it with confidence.*

4   *Walk in the hills with no regard to time.*

5   *Relax with who I am; revive my banter, laugh freely with friends.*

6   *Spend more time — fun time — with my family.*

7   *Begin my new career path. Trust it, be true to myself and bold with my voice.*

8   *Find peace in my home — if not in the one where I live, then in a new one.*

9   *Explore more of the west coast of Scotland.*

10   *Get a dog.*

11   *Believe in my talent to draw; lose myself in it, use it to relax.*

12   *Fulfil my dream to travel to the Maldives and swim with manta rays.*

13   *Jump out of a plane.*

14   *Walk the West Highland Way.*

15   *When I feel the urge for a spontaneous road trip, jump in Rocky and go.*

16   *Return to Croatia and breathe in the beauty of the Dalmatian Coast.*

17   *Work with or help promote cancer causes like Marie Curie and Maggie's Centres.*

18   *Take that longed-for trip to Italy.*

19   *Rekindle my love of mountain biking.*

20   *Ask five people close to me to suggest a new experience I could try. Pick one and do it. Perhaps do all.*

John

He is a perfectly tailored black wool coat, luxuriously woven, slightly scratchy, worn at the cuffs, not a speck of fluff, brightly polished buttons, lived-in but enduringly smart.

He is a Land Rover, battered by adventure, excited by impossible terrain, lovingly repaired, full of cranky old parts but always reliable, hurtling through clouds of angry black smoke.

He is a thistle, distinctive, handsome, proud and prickly. A reminder of hard-fought battles through treacherous glens, a symbol of patriotism, of brothers in arms.

He is Laphroaig whisky, sensually engaging, warmly peaty, bites of spice, and an age of stories. Persuasive but always a lingering hangover.

He is a rip-roaring sunrise on a biting, clear blue day when the clouds have not woken and the sun is preparing to riot.

He is blue, of sea and sky, of hypnotic depth, of a troubled unknown. True to the elements, vulnerable yet powerful, an energy alight with life at its fullest.

He is a Munro, intimidating but intriguing, imposing and respected, a challenge to all who love him.

He is a car horn, offensive but well meaning. To the ignorant, a jolt into action and awareness. To those he loves, his noise is protection, his message 'live in the moment'.

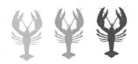

what I wish we had learned earlier

Each of us different, each cancer different, each of us at a different stage in our experience. Some happy outcomes, some tragic outcomes, a world of possibilities in between. I can only know what did and did not work for John and me as a couple, and for me alone. I share the things we wish we had discovered earlier as I'm aware from speaking to others that there are patches of common ground and that by talking about these we may feel less alone as we set tentative foot upon them.

Accept the help that is there as soon as you can
I make this plea to anyone who has been diagnosed with cancer and to those people closest to them. There are dedicated people who have the knowledge, experience and instincts to make it easier for you to live with cancer. Advice on practical, medical, emotional and financial matters really is only a phone call or visit away. Maggie's Centres, Marie Curie and Macmillan are only some of the crucial organisations that exist to help you through this. We were too proud and scared to go sooner, yet when we

finally accepted their help it allowed us to breathe again. You'll find a list of useful contacts at the end of this section.

If you are a carer, close friend or relative of someone with cancer, be informed

Gain knowledge about the type of cancer involved and the benefits and side effects of proposed treatments. Understand how the cancer and treatments may affect your loved one physically, mentally and emotionally. By keeping informed I was more aware of how John felt at different times of his illness, I was better able to understand what the consultants and doctors told us, more equipped to ask the right questions, to spot symptoms and side effects.

I don't suggest forcing someone to talk about his or her cancer diagnosis or treatment, absolutely not. I suggest that by accessing the vast amount of information available on cancer you will be better able to judge when someone with cancer may need emotional or physical support. An intuitively timed offer of a chat, a lift to hospital appointments, some grocery shopping can make a big difference without creating feelings of interference or pressure.

Be sensitive

Men and women, different personalities, will react in different ways to diagnosis. Pride, the fear of losing one's physical independence or a change to normal roles in work or in the family home, a reduction in social activities, a change in appearance can all affect how someone may react to offers of help. For the carer, a fear of being unable to cope with new pressures – practical, emotional, financial – may take its toll on their health too. If you're on the outside of their situation looking in, carefully consider life in their shoes before deciding how best to help them.

Make the most of appointments with your medical team

John and many others have told me that they 'switch off' during consultations, especially if they are hearing bad news. After the first few words the brain protects the heart, and concentration – let alone memory – is difficult. I began taking a note pad to appointments so that I could summarise what was being said and later repeat it to John. I also discovered that some doctors and hospitals are happy for you to record your consultation. Before appointments we would discuss what John's main concerns and questions were; again I'd write them down so that I could make sure we covered them all. John was never one to be quiet in business and social meetings, yet in consultations about his cancer he would often say very little. He was happier if I took it all in during the appointment and then we would go over it together later at home. If there were still questions unanswered, we would do some research and then ask our cancer care nurse or staff at Maggie's Centre for clarification.

It helped the medical team if we updated them properly on John's health. When we were both tired and often shrugging things off, we invariably missed important alarm bells. I began noting down changing symptoms or side effects of medication and treatment so that I could recall them to our doctors. The more aware you are of the changing condition, the more clearly you articulate your updates and questions, and the easier it is for the medical team to help you.

Dismiss the notion of 'fighting' the cancer

The cancer is there, always. Even if you are recovering or in remission, it lingers in the subconscious being. In reality it's part of us, our own cells. It feels like a bully of a houseguest intent on disrupting our lifestyle, but fighting with it, fighting with ourselves, or fighting with each other only saps essential energy and feeds the disease. We accepted that there was something (with a lot of baggage) in our house to work around, and we needed to change the way we did some things in order to maintain John and Rose's space. Eventually, we willingly changed our lives to ensure we had the time needed to keep the houseguest calm and under control. By working with it, by allowing it to be part of our routine, we managed to get time on our own.

Break down the walls of social and cultural discomfort

Let's be honest, in our society we are not very open about cancer. We may see media stories of famous people surviving or dying of cancer, of scientific advances, of charity events to raise awareness and funds, but are we really equipped to talk openly to people who are diagnosed with cancer? At work, in social situations, the very word is enough to send people into an uncomfortable scurry away, leaving the person who is talking about cancer twisted up in clumsy retorts and inappropriate humour in an attempt to ease the discomfort of everyone around them. We avoid the gaze of someone in a wheelchair, of someone with no hair, eyebrows and eyelashes. Why do we do this?

Some people around us were amazing – because they treated us as they always had done. If you've always had cheeky banter with someone then please don't stop that if they are suddenly diagnosed with cancer. Other people disappeared from our world. Perhaps it was fear of saying the wrong thing; perhaps it was fear of hearing about the reality of something they'd rather ignore. But, whether close or distant, most people who knew us felt worried and helpless.

We didn't help matters. We shut out most offers of help and brushed off the seriousness of our situation. If you can, try to be open with the people you care about. Explain what's going on, how you feel and how you would like to be treated and helped. An email or card may be easier than face to face, or hand people a book or website address where they can find out more. And let people help – what's a grocery shop, prepared meal, grass cut, house clean, lift to the hospital and back, school or club run, dog walk, new book or DVD between friends? It will ease your load and make them feel as if they are doing something to help. It doesn't mean you're failing or helpless, it doesn't mean they'll run away if they see your real hurt and frustration, it means you have good support around you. Cancer builds walls at speed if you allow it. Let people in and it will be harder for the cancer to pull you out of the world in which you feel real.

As for the situations where people watched me struggle to help John in and out of cars, through hospital doors, on and off planes, or ignored John as soon as he was confined to a wheel-chair, it's easy to get angry at this ignorance, but is it worth it if you know the people who matter are there to help you?

We never did master our infuriating pride and stubbornness. I really wish we had asked for and accepted more help than we did. Eventually people get fed up of offering help if they are constantly refused, and you may find you have no one there when you need help most. Not being open with people also meant that, after John died, no one around me really knew how much I had dealt with and why I was feeling as emotionally lost and physically exhausted as I was. Cancer and grief are crippling if you face them alone.

Plan time to feel alive

For a long time John and I lived in a blur of long working hours, perhaps trying to avoid facing the unwelcome houseguest, and dealing with one cancer trial after another. During these times we did not know whether the sun was shining, or whether either of us felt well or not. I certainly did not hear the birds sing or see the trees blossom. After far too long we acknowledged our blindness. We found our peace on holidays but also more regularly in the garden and out on walks. We rarely talked about the cancer during these times; we focused on each other and the moment we were in.

Be prepared for emergencies and for daily essentials

Type up a sheet summarising key medical history, current medications and treatments, the contact details of your oncologist and local GP. Keep this updated to ensure the treatment and medication notes are accurate. If you find yourself having to call out a doctor or an ambulance, or suddenly arriving at accident and emergency, hand over this sheet. Try to note down what led to the emergency, any changes you noticed in the preceding hours. The faster you can give nurses and doctors the information they need, the faster you will receive the right help. And take along some of the medications – it can take a long time, too long, to order replacements through the in-house hospital pharmacy.

Make a list of all the emergency and out-of-hours numbers you may need at home. Add any useful medical notes on temperature guidelines or worrying side effects. Keep the copies somewhere you can get to them quickly.

If you end up being treated in more than one hospital don't presume your usual hospital knows what's going on. Make sure the hospitals are updating each other on recent developments. If you have a problem, speak up; it may be a case of missing paperwork or a forgotten phone message. Hospitals are too short staffed and too busy to notice, so you may need to speak up more than once to be heard.

If you are managing a lot of different medications it helps to prepare a daily timetable that you can print out. As you dispense each med, tick it off the rota. Note any changes in symptoms, eating habits or bodily functions within the time slots.

Set your daily routine around the medical requirements so that you leave enough time for them, plus preparing meals, helping with washing, dressing and so on. If you're working at the same time, try to separate the two activities as much as possible. If you're handing over to a day nurse when you leave in the morning, update them thoroughly on changes during the night and any new symptoms you're keeping an eye on.

Give yourself the time you need to do each task, even if it means putting off visitors. After operations and as John's health deteriorated, my morning ritual of giving John meds, helping him to wash, dress and eat, took a couple of hours before we even began the day in other people's eyes. We learned to protect the time John needed to do each task comfortably.

I structured the day around medications and eating times and would timetable in a couple of hours when John and I were alone without visitors or medical people and when I wasn't doing tasks. We would go out together away from all the noise and just enjoy being us again. This became an incredibly special time for us but it did not happen unless we allocated it the same importance as medical visits.

Set boundaries for communication with family and friends

Keeping family and friends updated about how things are, especially at operation or treatment times, can be exhausting. It's natural for people to worry and to be absorbed in their own feelings, forgetting that you are dealing with many other people alongside them. I took ibuprofen daily to help with the pain in my right wrist and fingers – from texting so much.

Initially we tried to respond to everyone individually but this became impossible. I began to send out daily group texts to our family and friends summarising how John was. Gradually people realised I'd keep them updated as much as possible and they would wait for the daily or weekly update. If you feel bombarded explain to people that you need to update them on a group basis for a while whether via text, email or Facebook. If you're too tired to talk on the phone, say so. I sacrificed my own rest and many meals to respond to others. For our own sanity and welfare we needed to set manageable boundaries.

When we were told John was terminally ill, the demands of everyone around us were one of the hardest aspects to deal with. I know this sounds harsh, but it's true.

Trying to look after John and manage the enormous responsibilities of the situation we were in, while dealing with endless questions, other people's upset, politely serving coffee and biscuits and buoying conversation when I could see John was tiring, became too much. At one point it got so bad that we considered moving out to a rented holiday cottage for a few weeks. We are not alone in this; I know from Macmillan and Marie Curie nurses that many people really suffer because of such pressure. Fortunately our medical carers noticed how bad things had become and helped us to manage the situation more sensibly.

The patient's energy levels and comfort are the priorities so plan essential needs first: medicines, meals, doctor/nurse visits, personal care, rest periods. Remember that simple things like washing and dressing or moving rooms take much longer. Plan time to do it safely and comfortably. What does the person you love want to do... really want to do? Whatever it is, make sure they have the time to do it. Then – only then – commit to visitors, and when you do, ask people to be aware of signs that the 'patient' is tiring. Agree a 'secret signal' with your loved one so that you know when it's time to encourage guests to leave. Limit personal visits to times that suit you, and not every day. Cancel if either one of you is unwell, and politely ask that if your visitors have any colds or viruses they postpone their visit until they are well.

Be open minded about the hospice
The hospice is a place of highly trained people who can provide extra care when you need it. It's not a place focused on death, it's a safe haven designed to give you the best quality of life according to your own wishes.

Hospices offer physical, practical, emotional and spiritual care for the person with cancer and the people close to them. We found so much more than we expected. I felt enormous relief once we were under the care of the hospice – a place filled with light and peace where the doctors and nurses had the expertise and authority to administer medication to finally bring John's pain and symptoms under control. There were also social and occupational advisors, physiotherapists, chaplains and complementary therapists, all of them focused on helping John to achieve the best quality of life, in the way that he wanted, for as long as possible.

If you are the carer, take time out

If you're the carer, ask for cover occasionally. Speak to your doctor and the various cancer care organisations about how best to do this. It may be possible to get nursing cover for a few hours a week, a day or overnight. Remember that family and friends may not be permitted to administer strong and complicated medications, or may not feel comfortable being responsible in this way. Seek professional care where you can.

It's very easy to end up working, caring for your loved one and nothing else, but if you become ill you will be unable to care for them. As John said to me, he needed me to be well or he could not continue to live at home. I found it very hard to take time out without worrying but even an hour occasionally to go for a walk, get my sore neck and back treated, or my hair done, helped recharge me a little.

I also found that when I was at work I would overcompensate for the time I spent caring for John. I worked too hard and too long, skipping lunches and breaks as a way to lessen my worry and guilt. Cancer can happen to anyone, so you need to learn to trust that other people will understand; talk to your bosses and HR about what's happening and clarify their expectations.

It's important to find time to breathe. I did so by going to Maggie's Centre group sessions every few weeks. There I felt understood and supported.

Remember yourself

You become 'the patient' or 'the carer'. Necessity and routine can conspire to make you feel this way. Who were you before you became the patient or the carer? In a way, the cancer helped John remember who he was, not the guy too young to die from bladder cancer, not the financial advisor, not the invincible proud bloke from Fife, but John. I on the other hand totally forgot myself. I lived purely to make John better. I did not help John or myself by forgetting who Rose is.

If the worst happens, take your time, don't fight the loss

If you lose someone you love, go back to the start of this list: accept the help that's there as soon as you can. Until John died I did not truly appreciate grief's ability to absolutely consume a person. I will not lie: it never goes away, but you get used to it being a permanent part of you and slowly find ways to settle into your new being. I view it as my other uninvited houseguest and – as with cancer – I found it makes you feel unbearably uncomfortable in your own home, until you stop fighting it.

acknowledgements

Ok, so I didn't have much choice: write the book or break the promise I made to a man I love and respect, to a man alight in his last days. I'm not going to thank John for committing me to these pages as it's been an exhausting slog each muddy step of the way. And I'm a deeply private person so writing this book has been like me tackling Everest, barefoot. But John loved to make things mischievously difficult – often for one's own good – and I do thank him for that. And of course I'm happy to feel the relief and satisfaction gained only after pushing the mind and body somewhere uncomfortable before returning them to the hug of a hot bath, fresh home-cooked grub and a large glass of Sauvignon Blanc, which I currently glug to help me through these acknowledgements. Here goes.

John hid the extent of his pain from those closest to him. We were guilty of 'putting on a show' much of the time; our way to battle on regardless of the realities chasing us and those we loved. I am very aware that the honesty with which I've written about the effect of cancer on John has been deeply shocking and upsetting to those who loved him, and is especially painful for his two daughters whom he adored. The devastating loss of their father and knowing about the torments he endured cannot be softened by even those closest to them. John's hope was that his pain would not be forgotten by the medical community, cancer care organisations or policy makers; his story a lesson in the critical importance of a strong medical, psychological and practical network for those with cancer and those closest to them. I thank John's daughters for their courage in considering the book before it was printed. They were central figures in John's life but deserve their privacy and space and for this reason some names have been omitted or changed.

On a couple of occasions I do not name individuals because their actions and our subsequent upset were a moment in time and not to be held up as a judgement of their normal behaviour.

The charities...

I have chosen to support Maggie's Cancer Caring Centres and Marie Curie Cancer Care by making a donation from the sale of each book — and with my words of gratitude, which really do not go far enough to convey how truly remarkable and crucial both organisations are. Their people make it easier for anyone with or affected by cancer to see and feel life as a greater presence than the disease.

My friends at Maggie's: it's been a pleasure to work with you on the book and other publicity. For your help and support, I thank Elspeth Salter, Andy Anderson, Lisa Munden, Laura Lee, Sam Booth. At Marie Curie my thanks go to Dr David Oxenham, Paul Thompson, David Grout and Fiona Bushby.

The budding supporters...

Crucial in my tentative journey from heart to print were Stuart Delves, Jamie Jauncey and all the Dark Angels from Toftcombs, October 2010. Thank you for giving me the confidence to tell this story. If you missed that chapter, fear not: Dark Angels are not some underhand cult that took advantage of my grieving state. They are 'the business' when it comes to writing: inspirational mentors and courses that help people find their voice and sing humanity through each sentence.

The facts and forewords...
When I began piecing together the full story my memory did not gift me all the medical detail I desired, so sincere thanks to Duncan McLaren and Elliot Longworth for helping to fill in the gaps.

This book is a 'delicate' item to place – supportive to some, frightening to others – so I am humbly grateful for the experienced and wise words of Dr Elspeth Salter and Professor Marie Fallon to help position this book effectively and appropriately.

The first readers...
Those poor souls who were handed a hefty, raw manuscript full of typos, not to mention the deliberate angst and emotion, and asked: 'Is this any good?' What a question to ask; after all, I'd been through a spell of very bad luck, so telling me my hard work was flawed would not be easy. Thank you Stuart Delves, Andy Anderson, Elspeth Salter, Duncan McLaren, Marie Fallon, Peter Kravitz, Angus Ogilvy, Jamie Jauncey and John Beaton for constructive, directional feedback which fuelled my resolve to get this book out there, no matter what. And, John, I must mention you again as you probably have no idea just how much your help has meant to me: from professional advice to personal opinion. How unfair it is that you can relate to my words so deeply.

The serious business of publishing...
Not being a celebrity of A-list or even Z-list status, a cool cook, a quirky fiction spinner, a crime mastermind, a rogue politician, a self-help guru or a natural world navigator, I knew getting published would be difficult. I was wrong; it was soul-testingly difficult. A memoir by an unknown author, full of brutal honesty about a sensitive subject, in an unhappy economic and social climate is a 'risk' to any publisher. I'm lucky: my manuscript hit the desks of some open-minded, smashing folks. Even if they couldn't help, they pointed me in the right direction: John Beaton (again many thanks), Heather Holden-Brown, Jonathan Dimbleby, Jamie Jauncey, Sally Polson, Liffy Grant, and Marion Sinclair of Publishing Scotland – who led me to Sara:

Sara Hunt of Saraband Books. Sara of technology, history and trees, of the arts, mythology and bees... of the open heart and mind to agree to publish this book. You get it, all of it, you really do. I thank you for feeling the words and sharing the hope – and for steering me and this wayward book in the right direction.

Sincere thanks to David McKie of Levy & McRae for your invaluable legal advice and your personal support and encouragement for the book.

To Mairi Sutherland, caring editor, thank you for your appreciation of my sometimes rogue style, your belief in the book, and your focused but gentle approach to tidying it up. It was never going to be easy for me to trust someone to edit 'Rose and John' yet you made the process a pleasure.

Then there's the rather splendid cover illustration – thank you to the talented and accommodating Mitch Blunt.

Family and friends of the patient and loyal kind...

Of course then there's my loyal, patient, oh so patient, family and friends, who have had to watch this bumbling recluse insist on completing an exhausting project 'no matter what'. I'm sorry guys; I know you're on my side, even though I'm a stubborn pain in the butt. I've had support, which I appreciate enormously, from a lot of people, but there are a few I wish to mention specifically.

Gill & Nik: what can I say, you guys have been in it with me for the long haul and it aint been all banoffee pie, scratch cards, hearts and flowers. I treasure that photo mug; it's the four of us at our finest!

Mum (and Suzie): thanks for the long, sometimes wet and windy, sometimes sunny and calm, walks where I could chat things through, regain some perspective and recharge body and mind. And thanks for understanding me chucking in a sensible job and prospects to write and do lots of hippy stuff instead.

Kelly: high heels and champagne, to hair nets, custard tarts and plastic shoe covers. No one can say we haven't adapted to circumstances?! You are a rock of the sparkly kind. I know we reside in slightly different landscapes currently but the treasure is to be found in the middle ground where we can always don our jammies and comfort socks and 'laugh until our faces hurt'.

Paul: now that I've forgiven you for pouring a glass of wine into the pink laptop and almost halting the book altogether, there's so much to thank you for. The infuriating practical and technological stuff, the 'John chats', our chats, the road trips, but high-fiving an Amur tiger and stroking a bumble bee for the first time is just hard to beat.

J.A.: I know that reading details of your brother's pain must have been deeply upsetting. Thank you for your wise words, genuine support and encouragement.

Mighty Mike: have you any idea how much you have helped me deal with all 'the practical stuff' and therefore given me half a chance of writing this book? John would be so glad you are there for me, as I am. Thanks, thanks, thanks.

Beautiful Jen and your magical yurt: tears of sadness and of laughter but all of the healing kind. Thanks for sharing your twinkling serenity and fertile energy so that I could make this book a reality.

And dearest Darshi: a cheeky nod and wink to you for setting alight the exit sign at the zoo – I'm hurrying slowly headed for nowhere.

To end, I acknowledge some people who have been 'left out' of this book but who stood by me in a much more meaningful way than they needed to. For being friends not just colleagues, for caring words and distracting banter: the 'old team' at Scottish Widows. And 'P' and 'GT': thank you for standing by me and not strangling me, I know it can't have been easy.

And finally, with the strength and integrity of a truly great man in my mind:

> *Cherish the company of people who bring truth to your time and who help you to live life as if the end is nowhere in sight.*

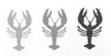

useful contacts

Maggie's Cancer Caring Centres

Maggie's is an organisation that creates places providing the emotional, practical and social support that people with cancer need. Designed by industry-leading architects, our Centres are warm, friendly and informal places full of light and open space with a big kitchen at their heart. They provide a peaceful space to absorb the information you're inevitably bombarded with and help to relieve the stress of having cancer. Maggie's wants to make the biggest difference personally to people with cancer at a scale that can make the most significant difference nationally.

General enquiries Maggie's Centres, 1st Floor,
One Waterloo Street, Glasgow G2 6AY
Email enquiries@maggiescentres.org
Tel 0300 123 1801
www.maggiescentres.org
Maggie Keswick Jencks Cancer Caring Centres Trust (Maggie's) is a registered charity, No. SC024414

Marie Curie Cancer Care

Marie Curie Cancer Care is a UK charity dedicated to the care of people with terminal cancer and other illnesses. We are best known for our network of 2,000 Marie Curie Nurses, who work in the homes of terminally ill patients across the UK, providing practical care and support.

Our nine Marie Curie Hospices across the UK provide expert care and the best quality of life for people with cancer and other illnesses.

We are the biggest provider of hospice beds outside the NHS, and we are expanding outpatient and day services at all our hospices. All our services are always free to patients and their families, thanks to the generous support of the public. We fund our nursing services and hospices in 50/50 partnership with the NHS.

Marie Curie Cancer Care, 89 Albert Embankment,
    London SE1 7TP
Tel 0800 716 146 (Monday to Friday, 9.00 am to 5.30 pm)
www.mariecurie.org.uk
Charity Reg No 207994 (England & Wales), SCO38731 (Scotland)

Dimbleby Cancer Care

Charity & Research Office
4th Floor Management Offices, Bermondsey Wing,
    Guy's Hospital, Great Maze Pond, London SE1 9RT
Tel 020 7188 7889
www.dimblebycancercare.org

Dimbleby Cancer Care Drop-in Centre — Guy's Hospital
Ground Floor, Tabard Annexe (formerly New Guy's House) within
    Clinical Oncology Outpatients, Guy's Hospital,
    Great Maze Pond, London SE1 9RT
Tel 020 7188 7188 / 5918

Dimbleby Cancer Care Drop-in Centre — St Thomas' Hospital
Lower Ground Floor, Lambeth Wing (just outside Clinical
    Oncology), St Thomas' Hospital,
    Westminster Bridge Road, London SE1 7EH
Tel 020 7188 5918

Macmillan Cancer Support

Practical, medical and financial support for people affected by cancer.
89 Albert Embankment, London SE1 7UQ
Tel 020 7840 7840 (head office)
Fax 020 7840 7841
Support line 0808 808 00 00
www.macmillan.org.uk

Cancer Research UK
National office
Cancer Research UK Angel Building, 407 St John Street,
London EC1V 4AD
Tel 0300 123 1861 (supporter services)
Tel 020 7242 0200 (switchboard)
Fax 020 3469 6400
www.cancerresearchuk.org

Children with Cancer
51 Great Ormond Street, London WC1N 3JQ
Tel 020 7404 0808
Fax 020 7404 3666
www.childrenwithcancer.org.uk

Clic Sargent – for Children with Cancer
Horatio House, 77–85 Fulham Palace Road, London W6 8JA
Tel 0300 330 0803 (head office); 0141 572 5700 (Scotland office)
www.clicsargent.org.uk

Everyman
An appeal of the Institute of Cancer Research to raise money for
research into prostrate and testicular cancer
The Institute of Cancer Research, 123 Old Brompton Road,
London SW7 3RP
Tel 020 7153 5375
Fax 020 7153 5313
www.everyman-campaign.org

Orchid
Support and information for people affected by or interested in
male-specific cancers.
St Bartholomew's Hospital, London EC1A 7BE
Monday to Friday 9.00am – 5.30pm
Tel 020 3465 5766
Fax 020 7600 1155
www.orchid-cancer.org.uk

Teenage Cancer Trust
3rd floor, 93 Newman Street, London W1T 3EZ
Tel 020 7612 0370
www.teenagecancertrust.org

ME association
Information, support and practical advice for people, families and carers affected by ME, CFS and PVFS.
7 Apollo Office Court, Radclive Road, Gawcott, Bucks MK18 4DF
Tel 01280 818964
www.meassociation.org.uk

Carers UK
Information and advice about caring and practical and emotional support for carers.
Tel 020 7378 4999 (England); 02920 811 370 (Wales);
0141 445 3070 (Scotland); 02890 439 843 (Northern Ireland)
Adviceline 0808 808 7777 (check website for opening hours)
www.carersuk.org

Carers Direct
Free, confidential information and advice for carers.
Tel 0808 802 0202
www.nhs.uk/carersdirect

CRUSE Bereavement Care
Unit 01, One Victoria Villas, Richmond TW9 2GW
Helpline 0844 477 9400
www.crusebereavementcare.org.uk

Winston's Wish
The largest provider of services to bereaved children, young people and their families in the UK
3rd Floor, Cheltenham House, Clarence Street,
    Cheltenham GL50 3JR
Helpline 08452 03 04 05
www.winstonswish.org.uk